# SpringerBriefs in Ethics

*SpringerBriefs in Ethics* envisions a series of short publications in areas such as business ethics, bioethics, science and engineering ethics, food and agricultural ethics, environmental ethics, human rights and the like. The intention is to present concise summaries of cutting-edge research and practical applications across a wide spectrum.

*SpringerBriefs in Ethics* are seen as complementing monographs and journal articles with compact volumes of 50 to 125 pages, covering a wide range of content from professional to academic. Typical topics might include:

- Timely reports on state-of-the art analytical techniques
- A bridge between new research results, as published in journal articles, and a contextual literature review
- A snapshot of a hot or emerging topic
- In-depth case studies or clinical examples
- Presentations of core concepts that students must understand in order to make independent contributions

Gabriel Andrade

# Trolleyology in Medicine

How the Trolley Problem Sheds Light
on Medical Ethics

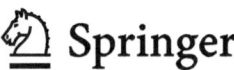 Springer

Gabriel Andrade
College of Medicine
Ajman University
Ajman, United Arab Emirates

ISSN 2211-8101 ISSN 2211-811X (electronic)
SpringerBriefs in Ethics
ISBN 978-3-031-72805-1 ISBN 978-3-031-72806-8 (eBook)
https://doi.org/10.1007/978-3-031-72806-8

This Springer imprint is published by the registered company Springer Nature Switzerland AG
The registered company address is: Gewerbestrasse 11, 6330 Cham, Switzerland

If disposing of this product, please recycle the paper.

# Introduction

In recent decades, Western nations have been experiencing what commentators now call the "culture wars." This is an ideological confrontation that pits various groups in an attempt to impose worldviews and specific values on society. The terminology for this phenomenon arose in 1870s Germany when the government and the Catholic Church were at odds in deciding who ought to control education and the appointment of clergy. At the time, journalists referred to that struggle as *Kulturkampf* (cultural struggle). Ever since the English translation has stuck, and the culture wars occupy a central role in contemporary society.

Whereas the original *Kulturkampf* was mostly about educational administration, the current culture wars encompass a wide variety of issues. Gay marriage, immigrants' rights, gender equality, racism, and secularism, amongst many others, elicit heated debates and cultural anxieties. Not surprisingly, they have increasingly become central topics in political campaigns throughout democratic nations.

Issues in medical ethics have been equally important in these culture wars. To the extent that they intersect with aspects of women's rights (as in abortion), or they pose a challenge to long-held assumptions about the sacredness of life (as in euthanasia), discussions about medical ethics are as relevant as ever in contemporary society. Furthermore, as humanity experienced its first pandemic in the age of social media and the internet, new challenges in medical ethics had to be addressed by the population at large, and not simply by medical practitioners and patients, as it was more customary in previous times.

Ever since Hippocrates formulated his famous oath for physicians, medical practitioners have reflected upon the principles that guide sound moral medical practice. Countless volumes have been dedicated to determining what those principles are, and how they apply to specific situations that are likely encountered by doctors on a frequent basis.

Yet, as medicine evolves, so do ethical challenges to the medical profession. The abstract principles that were traditionally established in previous times are still very relevant, but the complexities of modern times call for a reevaluation of many long-held assumptions. In this endeavor, the relevance of moral intuitions comes to the fore.

Ethicists have long discussed the value of intuition in moral judgment. Intuition may help individuals perceive and recognize moral aspects of particular situations; it can alert us to instances of harm, injustice, or moral conflict, prompting further reflection and deliberation. Likewise, intuition can shape how we perceive and interpret moral information, to the extent that it filters our understanding of a situation, highlighting certain aspects while downplaying or disregarding others.

Whatever intuitive principles are applied to moral reasoning in medicine, they must be sufficiently sound so as to have universal application. For that reason, in testing moral intuitions, it is important to appeal to scenarios that go beyond the usual realms of ethical reflection in medicine. Trolley scenarios can be very useful in this regard.

Thought experiments have a long history in philosophy, but it was not until the mid-twentieth century that ethicists realized their enormous potential to clarify intuitions and sharpen moral reasoning. Philippa Foot's seminal work explored how specific situations can shed light on all aspects of ethics. In her original formulation, a trolley driver must decide whether it is acceptable to divert a trolley to kill one person in order to save five.

Foot opened some floodgates of moral reasoning, as her original musings about trolley scenarios gave way to a plethora of variations to further test ethical intuitions. This has occasioned the rise of a particular field of ethics that some have even styled as "trolleyology." Most philosophical activity on trolleyology pertains to the intricacies of moral decision-making in the abstract, as trolley scenarios help us refine relevant moral principles to be applied in everyday moral decision-making.

Yet it becomes clear that trolleyology is also very relevant in applied ethics. This is especially the case in the medical realm. For example, how can we determine the moral adequacy of euthanasia? Partly, we can answer that question by establishing if there is a difference between doing and allowing. In turn, we can think about whether a driver's decision to divert a trolley to avoid killing five is equivalent to a bystander's decision to do the same.

Despite the obvious overlap between trolleyology and medical ethics, no book has been written specifically mapping out this connection. The present volume seeks to fulfill that task. The book is structured around three chapters, and each chapter will focus on a central topic of medical ethics: euthanasia, abortion, and public health. By way of introduction in each chapter, I will present a historical figure that has become central in the culture wars, related to each of the three main topics of discussion: Dr. Jack Kevorkian in the culture wars over euthanasia, Norma McCorvey in the culture wars over abortion, and Mary Mallon in the culture wars over public health. I will then examine many of the variations of the trolley dilemmas that shed light on these particularly contentious issues in medical ethics, as well as further moral reflections and thought experiments that serve as corollaries of trolleyology.

In exploring the intricate interplay between trolleyology and medical ethics, this book embarks on a pioneering journey. Just as the trolley dilemma illuminates the nuances of moral decision-making, so too does this volume seek to elucidate the moral landscape of medicine, offering insights that resonate far beyond the confines of the clinic. By weaving together the threads of ethical theory and real-world practice, we strive towards a deeper understanding of the ethical imperatives that shape our shared humanity.

# Contents

# Chapter 1
# Euthanasia

**Abstract** This chapter approaches Dr. Jack Kevorkian's legacy in the culture wars, by way of introduction to the moral complexities of euthanasia. In the outlook of most codes of medical ethics, euthanasia is morally acceptable, provided it is only done passively (i.e., solely withdrawing treatment). This stance is grounded in the moral difference between killing and letting die. Philipa Foot's original consideration of trolley scenarios was intended to support this distinction. However, a thought experiment by James Rachels challenges that distinction. Furthermore, a variation of the trolley scenario by Judith Jarvis Thomson suggests that, in some circumstances, killing one may be even preferable to letting five die. Despite these nuances, the distinction between doing and allowing harm may still be relevant, although that does not imply that euthanasia is morally unacceptable in every case. Ultimately, notions of compassion and autonomy do warrant the moral acceptability of euthanasia, albeit such decisions must be handled with care and on a case-by-case basis.

One of the most divisive figures in the culture war of the past three decades was Dr. Jack Kevorkian. A highly intelligent man, Kevorkian was a pathologist by training. From a very young age, he had a penchant for controversial ideas. As a teenager, he appealed to the so-called 'problem of evil' in order to deny the existence of God; being of Armenian descent, he could not come to terms with the idea that an omnipotent and benevolent God would not stop the Armenian genocide of the 1910s.

As a student, he embraced the prospect of using death row prisoners as subjects for human experiments: "I propose that a prisoner condemned to death by due process of law be allowed to submit, by his own free choice, to medical experimentation under complete anaesthesia (at the time appointed for administering the penalty) as a form of execution in lieu of conventional methods prescribed by law" [1]. This would not be his last controversy.

He would become especially notorious in the 1980s, when he advertised his practice in newspapers, as "death counselling" [2]. He then began to assist patients in pursuing their own death. This led to various criminal charges. He was tried in trial four times; he was acquitted in three of those instances, and one resulted in a

© The Author(s) 2024

G. Andrade, *Trolleyology in Medicine*, SpringerBriefs in Ethics,

https://doi.org/10.1007/978-3-031-72806-8_1

mistrial. Kevorkian was bold enough to allow the *60 Min* TV show to air footage of him administering lethal injections to one of his patients [3].

This ran counter to the ethical stance of the American Medical Association. They have issued the following statement: "Euthanasia is the administration of a lethal agent by another person to a patient for the purpose of relieving the patient's intolerable and incurable suffering. It is understandable, though tragic, that some patients in extreme duress—such as those suffering from a terminal, painful, debilitating illness—may come to decide that death is preferable to life. However, permitting physicians to engage in euthanasia would ultimately cause more harm than good. Euthanasia is fundamentally incompatible with the physician's role as healer, would be difficult or impossible to control, and would pose serious societal risks. Euthanasia could readily be extended to incompetent patients and other vulnerable populations. The involvement of physicians in euthanasia heightens the significance of its ethical prohibition. The physician who performs euthanasia assumes unique responsibility for the act of ending the patient's life" [4].

On the basis of this ethical stance, Kevorkian's medical license was revoked in 1991 [5]. Even without a license, he continued to assist patients in their desire to die, and he was finally convicted of second-degree homicide in 1999. He served a sentence of eight years.

Euthanasia remains a hotly contested topic in the public sphere. It is important to understand that in this regard, euthanasia is composed of two elements that must be carefully assessed: the act and the motive. The act refers to the physical action or procedure carried out to bring about the death of a person who is terminally ill or suffering unbearably. This could involve administering a lethal dose of medication, removing life-sustaining treatment, or any other direct action that results in the person's death.

The motive, on the other hand, pertains to the underlying reason or intention behind the act of euthanasia. Motives can vary widely and may include compassion for the suffering individual, a desire to relieve their pain and distress, respect for their autonomy and wishes, or even personal or societal beliefs about the value of life and the right to die with dignity.

Distinguishing between the act and motive is important because laws regarding euthanasia often focus on the act itself and whether it is permissible under certain circumstances, such as when the patient is terminally ill and has made a voluntary and informed decision to end their life. Motives may also be considered in legal proceedings to determine the intention behind the act and whether it was carried out with malicious intent or genuine compassion.

But these two dimensions also go beyond legal aspects. Ethical debates surrounding euthanasia often delve into questions of motive, exploring whether the act is driven by a genuine concern for the well-being of the patient or by other factors such as financial considerations, pressure from family members, or societal attitudes towards disability and illness.

Most approaches to the euthanasia debate are overly simplistic, and some clarifications are also needed. First, it is important to distinguish various types of euthanasia, classified along two axes: level of participation provided by the healthcare practitioner, [6] and level of consent provided by the patient [7].

In passive euthanasia, a healthcare practitioner may withhold or withdraw medical treatment or life-sustaining measures with the intention of allowing a patient to die naturally. This does not involve taking direct action to cause the patient's death but rather ceasing interventions that are keeping the patient alive.

Various such procedures are common in this regard. For example, there may be withholding of life-sustaining treatment; this involves refraining from initiating or continuing medical interventions that are aimed at prolonging life. Decisions not to start or to discontinue artificial ventilation, cardiopulmonary resuscitation (CPR), [8] or dialysis for a terminally ill patient, are usually considered part of this endeavor.

Likewise, there may be withdrawal of Artificial Nutrition and Hydration (ANH). In some cases, patients may receive food and fluids through tubes, such as a naso-gastric tube or a gastrostomy tube; withdrawing these forms of artificial nutrition and hydration can lead to a natural decline in the patient's condition and eventual death [9]. Perhaps more commonly, physicians may discontinue medications that are not providing significant benefit to the patient or that are causing undue suffering; this could include stopping antibiotics for infections or medications used to control symptoms such as pain or nausea.

Furthermore, in cases where a patient is experiencing severe pain or distress that cannot be adequately relieved by other means, palliative sedation may be used. This involves administering medication to induce a state of sedation, potentially hastening the patient's death as a secondary effect of the treatment [10]. As we shall see in the next chapter, this type of procedure is sometimes confused with active euthanasia, but there are important moral principles that establish a differences between deliberately killing a patient, and simply administer substances to relieve pain, in the foreknowledge that a side effect will be the death of the patient.

In contrast, active euthanasia involves taking deliberate and affirmative action to end a person's life, usually through the administration of lethal substances or interventions. In this case, it is the direct act of causing death with the explicit intention of relieving suffering or pain. For example, active euthanasia may be carried out by administering a lethal injection or providing a lethal dose of medication to the patient. This was the type of procedure carried out by Dr. Kevorkian.

Other methods of active euthanasia have also been used in some instances. For example, physicians may assist patients in hastening their death, by providing medi-cation to end their life. This medication is typically self-administered by the patient after obtaining a prescription from a qualified healthcare provider [11]. This type of procedure implies providing a terminally ill or suffering individual with the means (such as medication) to end their own life, while the individual themselves admin-isters the lethal dose. This may involve prescribing or providing medication and ensuring that the patient understands how to use it effectively to bring about death.

Passive euthanasia is considered ethically acceptable by the American Medical Association and similar institutional bodies worldwide, provided the patient agrees to it. This stance relies on the importance of patient autonomy, as no patient can be forced to accept treatment without consent.

However, the question of consent is itself controversial. It has been traditionally stipulated that in the context of euthanasia, there must be some important elements so as to ensure that the decision is truly consented upon by the patient. First, the patient must possess decision-making capacity or competence, meaning they are able to understand relevant information about their medical condition, prognosis, and the implications of euthanasia [12]. They should be capable of weighing the risks and benefits of their decision and communicating their wishes clearly.

It is also of crucial importance to consider that the request for euthanasia must be voluntary and freely made by the individual without any external pressure, coercion, or manipulation from others. The individual must provide informed consent to undergo euthanasia, indicating that they have been fully informed about their medical condition, treatment options, prognosis, potential risks and benefits of euthanasia, and available alternatives. They should understand the nature of euthanasia and its irreversible consequences.

The request for euthanasia should be stable over time, indicating that the individual has carefully considered their options and has not made a hasty or impulsive decision. Healthcare providers should assess the consistency of the individual's request and ensure that it is not influenced by temporary factors such as depression, anxiety, or inadequate pain management. Furthermore, there should be no external influence, coercion, or undue pressure from others, including family members, healthcare providers, or caregivers, to pursue euthanasia [13]. Likewise, there should always be opportunities for the patients to reconsider their decision and explore alternative options, such as palliative care, pain management, hospice care, or psychological support.

In this context, it is important to keep in mind that totalitarian systems were eager to employ euthanasia procedures to get rid of undesirables in society, completely disregarding the ethical importance of informed consent in any medical procedure. For example, the Nazis implemented a program of involuntary euthanasia, known as the "T4 Program," as part of their eugenics policies aimed at "purifying" the German population [14]. The primary targets of this program were individuals with disabilities and mental illnesses. The Nazis believed that these individuals were a burden on society; they established several euthanasia centers across Germany and German-occupied territories during World War II, and individuals deemed "unworthy of life" (*lebensunwertes leben*) were systematically killed [15]. Patients were transported to the euthanasia centers under the guise of receiving medical treatment, and then they were killed using gas chambers disguised as showers [16].

Various historians assert that the T4 Program served as a precursor to the Holocaust, during which millions of Jews and other groups were systematically murdered [17, 18]. Needless to say, this program violated the fundamental human rights of individuals with disabilities and other targeted groups, as it denied them the right to life, autonomy, and dignity, treating them as inferior and unworthy of existence solely based on their perceived disabilities or illnesses. Of course, this is an extreme historical experience, but it is important to note that the T4 program began as a violation of patients' consent, and consequently, healthcare practitioners must take this aspect of medical practice very seriously.

However, there are some cases of euthanasia that, although not fully involuntary, cannot be properly called "voluntary" either. We have already established that voluntary euthanasia occurs when a competent individual makes a conscious and informed decision to end their own life with the assistance of a healthcare provider or another person. In contrast, the Nazis pursued involuntary euthanasia to the extent that patients' lives were ended against their wishes, without their consent, or despite their explicit refusal of euthanasia.

But there may be a third category that we may label "non-voluntary." This happens when a patient is unable to provide consent or express their wishes regarding end-of-life care, often due to unconsciousness, cognitive impairment, or being in a persistent vegetative state [19, 20]. In these cases, the decision to end the patient's life is made by others, such as family members, legal guardians, or healthcare providers, based on what they believe to be in the patient's best interests. This may occur in the context of patients in vegetative state that have not expressed their wishes regarding end-of-life care in an advance directive, and their family members, in consultation with healthcare professionals, decide to withdraw life-sustaining treatment. This type of procedure may give rise to ethical debates.

Consider, for example, the case of Terri Schiavo [21]. She was a woman in Florida who suffered severe brain damage and fell into a persistent vegetative state (PVS) in 1990. Her husband and legal guardian, Michael Schiavo, argued that she had expressed wishes not to be kept alive by artificial means in such a condition. Terri's parents, on the other hand, fought to keep her on life support. The case went to court, and it was decided that her feeding tubes would be removed, which led to her death. In this regard, this was a form of passive euthanasia, but because it was not fully consensual (the patient was in no capacity to fully agree to it), it aroused controversy [22].

As of now, consensual active euthanasia is allowed in some jurisdictions in the United States, provided it is in the form of self-administered Physician-Assisted Dying (PAD): Washington, Vermont, California, Colorado, District of Columbia, Hawaii, New Jersey, Maine, New Mexico and Montana. Active consensual euthanasia is also legal in Canada, some regions of Australia, Austria, Belgium, Finland, Germany, Luxembourg, the Netherlands, Spain, Switzerland and Colombia [23].

Although some caution must be kept, we may assume that there is a pattern to the places where euthanasia has been legalized. They tend to be countries with more liberal attitudes towards individual rights and autonomy, as sociological research shows that these societies prioritize individual autonomy and the right to make decisions about one's own life, including end-of-life decisions [24]. Likewise, countries with advanced healthcare systems often grapple with end-of-life care issues, including how to address severe suffering in terminally ill patients [25]. Furthermore, such countries tend to have higher levels of secularism, as religious objections to euthanasia, often based on the sanctity of life doctrine, can influence policy decisions in more religiously conservative societies [26]. Observers have also noted that legalization of euthanasia often occurs in countries with democratic governance systems where public opinion and societal values play a significant role in shaping legislation; [27] this allows for debates and discussions on the topic, leading to policy changes reflective of societal attitudes.

Another important pattern to be found in societies legalizing euthanasia is that they tend to have prominent human rights discourses [28]. Advocates for euthanasia often frame the issue in terms of human rights, emphasizing the right to die with dignity and the right to avoid unnecessary suffering; this discourse can gain traction in societies with strong human rights movements and legal frameworks.

According to opponents of euthanasia, passive euthanasia is acceptable but active euthanasia is unacceptable, because there is a fundamental difference between doing and allowing harm. Fiona Woolard provides an adequate summary of the doctrine upholding this difference: "The Doctrine of Doing and Allowing (DDA) states that, when other people are harmed because of the way we behave, it matters morally whether we have done harm or merely allowed harm. More precisely, doing harm is harder to justify than merely allowing harm. If jumping into the river to save Bob would cost you your life, it is permissible to allow him to drown but it is not permissible to push him into the river to save your own life. If you must choose between rescuing both Fred and Frieda from a fire and rescuing George, it is permissible to allow George to die so you can save a greater number, but it is not permissible to run over and kill George even if this is the only way to get to the others in time" [29].

As applied to the case of euthanasia, this corresponds with a difference between killing and letting die. This goes back to the very foundation of the original Hippocratic Oath, and its emphasis on *primum non nocere*—first doing no harm [30]. In one account, death is itself a harm, so it is not allowed for a physician to actively participate in the intentional death of a patient, even if that action may serve some noble purpose [31].

But the doctrine distinguishing between doing and allowing harm (or between killing and letting die) is far from universally accepted, and critics of the status quo in euthanasia frequently claim that the doctrine is obsolete. As it happens, this discussion can be better understood by considering the original trolley problem.

## The Original Trolley Problem

As mentioned in the Introduction, the starting point of the trolley problem was Philippa Foot. In her seminal 1967 paper, "The Problem of Abortion and the Doctrine of the Double Effect", Foot's intention was to scrutinize the doctrine of double effect, "which is invoked by Catholics in support of their views on abortion but supposed by them to apply elsewhere" [32]. According to the doctrine of double effect, some actions that cause harm are allowed, provided the harms are only unintended but foreseen consequences of the actions, and the harms are proportional to the original aim of the action. As per this doctrine, abortion is not ethically permissible, because it seeks to directly cause a harm (i.e., the death of the fetus), and the harm is not merely foreseen.

Catholics have traditionally embraced this doctrine to account for the moral difference between a fetus' death as a result of a hysterectomy, and a fetus' death as a result of abortion. Abortion involves the deliberate termination of a pregnancy, which, in most cases, results in the death of the fetus. Under the doctrine of double effect, abortion is morally unacceptable because its primary intent is to end the life of the fetus, and the harmful consequence (the death of the fetus) is directly intended.

In contrast, a hysterectomy is a surgical procedure in which a woman's uterus is removed. This procedure can be performed for various medical reasons, including treating conditions such as uterine cancer, severe endometriosis, or life-threatening hemorrhaging during childbirth. As per the doctrine of double effect, a hysterectomy is morally acceptable when it is medically necessary to address a serious health issue or to save the life of the woman, even if results in the death of the fetus. In this case, the primary intent is a therapeutic one—to treat a medical condition or prevent a serious health risk. The secondary consequence, the death of the fetus, is not intended but rather an unfortunate outcome.

The key difference between abortion and a hysterectomy within the context of the doctrine of double effect is the primary intent of the action. Abortion is primarily intended to end a pregnancy, while a hysterectomy is primarily intended for medical treatment, such as removing a cancerous uterus.

But Foot was not persuaded that the doctrine of double effect made full sense. She was concerned about the impreciseness of intention. She thought there was a 'problem of closeness,' in the sense that it was not always possible to distinguish between intentions when agents carried on some actions. She invites us to consider this scenario: "A party of potholers have imprudently allowed the fat man to lead them as they make their way out of the cave, and he gets stuck, trapping the others behind him. Obviously the right thing to do is to sit down and wait until the fat man grows thin; but philosophers have arranged that floodwaters should be rising within the cave. Luckily (luckily?) the trapped party have with them a stick of dynamite with which they can blast the fat man out of the mouth of the cave. Either they use the dynamite or they drown. In one version the fat man, whose head is in the cave, will drown with them; in the other he will be rescued in due course. Problem: may they use the dynamite or not" [32]?

If they used the dynamite, they would intend the fat man's death. It would seem that under the doctrine of double effect, such an action is not allowed. But what if they claim that their intention was not to kill the fat man, but rather, simply to blow him to pieces, so as to make way for the explorers to escape?

In fact, in the context of medical ethics, some authors had pointed out that in instances such as euthanasia and abortion, the intended effect is not death itself, and therefore, the action would be allowed as per the doctrine of double effect. For example, H. L. A. Hart argued as follows: "if a woman is found to have cancer of the womb of which she will die unless the womb is removed, the surgeon may, according to Catholic doctrine, remove the womb with the foreseen consequence that the foetus dies. On the other hand, he is not permitted to perform a craniotomy killing an unborn child to save a woman in labour who would die if the head of the foetus is not crushed. Yet in such cases it could be argued that it is not the death of the foetus but its removal from the body of the mother which is required to save her life" [33]. As per this argument, the intention in abortion is not to kill the fetus, but simply to remove it from the woman's body, very much as the intention of the potholers is not to kill the fat man, but simply to blow him to pieces.

Foot concedes these explanations would be absurd, but she is quick to point out that if the doctrine of double effect were used, there would be "difficulty in explaining where the line is to be drawn" [32] as there may be cases in which it is not easy to separate between the foreseen act and the intended act; in some cases, "one is justified in bringing about knowingly what one could not directly intend" [32].

Foot was therefore seeking a moral principle that would provide firmer ground to separate acceptable from unacceptable actions. She introduces the following case: "Suppose that a judge or magistrate is faced with rioters demanding that a culprit be found for a certain crime and threatening otherwise to take their own bloody revenge on a particular section of the community. The real culprit being unknown, the judge sees himself as able to prevent the bloodshed only by framing some innocent person and having him executed" [32].

This is in fact a type of situation that has long been used against utilitarians. If, as utilitarians following Jeremy Bentham's famous dictum have it, "it is the greatest happiness of the greatest number that is the measure of right and wrong" [34] then it seems that there is no choice but to approve of the judge's plan. For, if the plan is brought to fruition, the wider community will be saved at the expense of one innocent man, and a greater number of lives will be preserved.

Some utilitarians have famously bitten the bullet in cases such as this and have agreed that maximizing utility (in this case, saving a greater number of lives) is the guiding principle. But Foot was not a utilitarian. She thought that it would be wrong to kill the innocent man, even if that saved a greater number of lives. Nevertheless, she did not endorse a blanket prohibition against killing. She acknowledged that sometimes, one is authorized to make decisions that entail killing someone, in order to save more. She thus presents the case of the tram, whence the trolly problem would be born. Foot asks us to imagine the "driver of a runaway tram which he can only steer from one narrow track on to another; five men are working on one track and one man on the other; anyone on the track he enters is bound to be killed" [32]. Foot acknowledges that in this case, the driver is justified in diverting the tram. His action results in the killing of one worker, but he is morally bound to do so, because by his very actions (having put the tram on its course previously), one person would die anyways. Given that saving five is better than saving one, there is justification to kill.

Foot wanted to know why it would be acceptable to kill one to save five in the tram case, but it would not be acceptable to kill the innocent man in order to save the community. She complemented that comparison with further cases from medical ethics. For example: "[why] do we not feel justified in killing people in the interests of cancer research or to obtain, let us say, spare parts for grafting on to those who need them? We can suppose, similarly, that several dangerously ill people can be saved only if we kill a certain individual and make a serum from his dead body" [32].

Foot pondered whether intention might be the response to her query. She considered whether establishing a difference between direct and oblique intention might solve the issue. The judge has the direct intention of killing the innocent man, whereas the driver only has the oblique intention of killing the man on the track. Again, as the doctrine of double effect would have it, the extent to which the effects are intended seems to count. But recall that in many cases intended effects and foreseen effects are too close.

Furthermore, Foot believed there were some cases in which intentions would clearly not be an adequate guide to determine the morality of the action. She advances yet another scenario that pertains to medical ethics: "there are five patients in a hospital whose lives could be saved by the manufacture of a certain gas, but that this inevitably releases lethal fumes into the room of another patient whom for some reason we are unable to move. His death, being of no use to us, is clearly a side effect, and not directly intended" [32].

In this case, the doctrine of double effect would authorize the administration of the gas. The death of the one patient is a lesser harm compared to the death of the five patients, and the death of the one patient is not intended; it is merely a side effect of the action. Foot believed that releasing the fumes would nevertheless be wrong, and counted this case as an illustration of why the doctrine of double effect is not an adequate guide to morality.

But it is far from clear that in this case, releasing the fumes is wrong. In fact, the administration of many treatments operates on this basis. Consider vaccines. The administration of vaccines at an early age helps prevent the deaths of millions of people. Vaccines are rigorously tested for safety and effectiveness before they are approved for use, and they go through multiple phases of clinical trials to assess their safety and efficacy. However, like all medical interventions, vaccines are not entirely without risk [35]. In rare cases, vaccines can cause adverse events, including serious ones. It's important to note that the risk of experiencing a serious adverse event from a vaccine is extremely low, and the benefits of vaccination far outweigh the risks for the vast majority of people. Yet, some harmful cases have indeed been reported, some of them fatal [36].

There are various types of risks associated with vaccines. Some individuals may experience allergic reactions to vaccine components, such as egg proteins (in certain vaccines) or other vaccine ingredients. Severe allergic reactions are very rare. For example, in rare cases, vaccines, such as the influenza vaccine, have been associated with an increased risk of Guillain-Barré Syndrome, a rare neurological disorder. There have also been extremely rare cases of blood clotting disorders associated with specific vaccines, like the Johnson & Johnson COVID-19 vaccine and the AstraZeneca COVID-19 vaccine. Furthermore, some vaccines, like the MMR (measles, mumps, and rubella) vaccine, have been associated with a slightly increased risk of febrile seizures in children, but these are generally not life-threatening. The oral polio vaccine (OPV) can, in very rare instances, lead to vaccine-associated paralytic polio.

All of these are unintended yet foreseen effects of vaccines, and they may even result in deaths. Whenever such deaths happen, one may well argue that such deaths are the result of the decision of introducing vaccines, so the victims of those side effects have been killed by the decision to introduce the vaccines. Yet no reasonable public health official would argue that it is better not to introduce the vaccines. The benefits outweigh the harms, and the harms are not intended.

Perhaps Foot's scenario of the fumes is not exactly analogous to the introduction of vaccines, as in the former, the patient who dies has no connection whatsoever to the fumes, whereas in the latter, the people who die as a result of vaccines do have a connection with the initial action, to the extent that they originally participated as beneficiaries of the vaccine. But we can still think of other situations in medical contexts that are closer to the fumes example, and yet, it would seem that there is moral authority to pursue the action. For example, for public health purposes, an area of a camp with radioactive waste disposal may be fenced, and if touched, this fence may emit mild electric charges. By keeping people off from this area, setting up the fence prevents many people from being exposed to radiation, and therefore, many lives are saved. However, one visitor from another country who is not prone to developing cancer, but who has some cardiovascular complications, may incidentally touch the fence, and as a result, may die. Again, in that case, even though the death of that person may be foreseen, it is still unintended, and given that a larger number of people are saved to the extent that they are kept away from the radioactive waste, it would be sensible to set up the fence, even with that acknowledged risk.

In any case, Foot insists that in the case of the fumes, there is no moral authority to release them. Even if the effect is unintended, in this case she does not accept the prospect of killing one in order to save five. But in the tram scenario, she does accept the prospect of killing one to save five. What, then, is the difference between both scenarios?

Foot argues that it depends on how the five die. If the dilemma is between killing one and killing five, then it is morally acceptable to kill, as in the case of the driver who diverts the tram. Furthermore, if the dilemma is between letting one die and letting five die then utilitarian calculations may be considered, and ultimately, one may choose the action that saves the greatest number of lives. Foot presents the following medical scenario in order to illustrate this point: "We are about to give a patient who needs it to save his life a massive dose of a certain drug in short supply. There arrive, however, five other patients each of whom could be saved by one-fifth of that dose. We say with regret that we cannot spare our whole supply of the drug for a single patient, just as we should say that we could not spare the whole resources of a ward for one dangerously ill individual when ambulances arrive bringing in victims of a multiple crash. We feel bound to let one man die rather than many if that is our only choice" [32].

Interestingly, some people have disagreed with this assessment of that scenario. For example, in a rejoinder to Foot's article, Elizabeth Anscombe argued as follows: "There seems to me nothing wrong with giving the single patient the massive dose and letting the others die, of with refusing to deprive the single patient of care necessary to keep him alive because the hands needed for that care could help in saving the many victims of an accident… It seems to me justifiable to say one can't spare those three people because of the job they are doing, if their work seems roughly as likely to save that one person as to save several to whose aid they could be called" [37]. Anscombe based her argument on the claim that neither of the patients are owed the drug (or the medical care), and nobody is harmed by being refused the drug. Consequently, there is no harm done in choosing to save one over choosing to save five, as none of the five are owed anything.

This is not a very persuasive line of reasoning. Numbers do not matter in all instances, but surely there is an imperative to, other things being equal, maximize the good we can do. Even if the patients are not owed anything, wasting scarce resources without attempting to maximize their usefulness is itself a moral failure. Indeed, this is the moral imperative in critical situations as per the triage system in medical ethics, [38] such as was implemented during the COVID-19 pandemic.

The triage system in medical ethics and practice is a method used to prioritize patients in emergency situations or when resources are limited. It helps healthcare professionals make decisions about who should receive medical treatment first based on the severity of their condition and the available resources. Triage is a critical component of disaster medicine and is also used in emergency departments during overcrowded or high-demand periods. Although the protocols and selection criteria may vary (I will expand on this in Chap. 3), in triage situations, patients are assessed to determine the urgency of their medical needs. This initial assessment is often performed by a nurse or healthcare provider. Afterwards, patients are assigned to different triage categories based on the severity of their condition. Triage decisions are then made based on the principle of maximizing overall benefit. In situations where resources are limited, the goal is to allocate resources to those who have the best chance of survival or recovery. This may entail abandoning the care of a patient in very bad condition in order to allocate resources for patients with higher probabilities of survival. Under these ethical presumptions, there is simply no space for Anscombe's argument. Patients in triage situations may not be owed medical attention per se, but certainly, the medical profession is committed to trying to make the best out of whatever resources are available.

Consequently, it is preferable to let one die instead of letting five die. But if the dilemma is between killing one and letting five die, then Foot argues that it is *not* morally acceptable to kill. In the case of the judge or the fumes in the hospital, not doing something leads to a greater number of deaths. But that greater number of deaths cannot be morally attributed to the person who refused to carry out the action, since that action itself results in death. Foot's point is that while we could be held responsible for things we fail to do, that responsibility can never be on the same par as the responsibility for the things we do.

Foot appealed to the difference between positive duties and negative duties. Negative duties are duties of non-interference or duties of restraint. These duties involve refraining from doing harm to others or preventing harm from occurring. Negative duties typically require inaction, such as not stealing, not lying, or not causing physical harm to someone. In essence, negative duties are obligations not to engage in certain harmful actions.

In contrast, positive duties are duties of action or duties to do something to benefit others. They involve taking affirmative steps to promote the well-being of others or to prevent harm. Positive duties could include helping those in need, providing aid, or fulfilling promises. These duties require proactive engagement and assistance.

This difference is reminiscent of Isaiah Berlin's distinction of positive and negative liberties. In his seminal work of political philosophy, "Two Concepts of Liberty", Berlin established two types of liberty [39]. Negative liberty, according to Berlin, is the absence of external interference or constraints on an individual's actions. It is the freedom from being coerced or hindered by others. Negative liberty is often associated with the idea of individual rights and the limitation of state power to interfere with personal choices and actions. Positive liberty, on the other hand, is the capacity or ability to act in accordance with one's own rational will. It implies self-realization and the freedom to achieve one's potential. Positive liberty may involve state intervention or social and economic conditions that enable individuals to pursue their goals.

While Berlin acknowledged that liberal regimes must find a proper balance between the two types of liberty, he was cautious about the potential dangers of positive liberty when taken to extremes, as it could lead to authoritarianism or paternalism, where the State or a collective decides what is in an individual's best interest. Admittedly, he did not explicitly say that negative liberties are of a higher order than positive liberties, but he did caution against the potential dangers of an unbalanced or extreme emphasis on positive liberty at the expense of negative liberty.

Foot argued for a similar approach in the balance of positive and negative duties. While acknowledging the importance of positive duties, she insisted that if they come into conflict, negative duties are more important than positive duties. Therefore, if in order to avoid letting five persons die, we must kill one person, then it is better to let the five persons die. Although inaction may be reprehensible in many cases, it is never as bad as actively doing something that brings about harm. Foot makes the case as follows: "if we are bringing aid... we must obviously rescue the larger rather than the smaller group. It does not follow, however, that we would be justified in inflicting the injury, or getting a third person to do so, in order to save the five... To refrain from inflicting injury ourselves is a stricter duty than to prevent other people from inflicting injury, which is not to say that the other is not a very strict duty indeed" [32].

It should be noted that Foot did not imply that positive duties are irrelevant. This is a point that must be emphasized in the context of medical ethics. Physicians have a duty to aid their patients, as the principle of beneficence establishes [40]. This is one of the fundamental ethical principles that guide healthcare professionals and institutions in their decisions and actions. Beneficence is often summarized as the principle of 'doing good' and refers to the obligation to promote the well-being and best interests of the patient. A physician is not entitled to refuse treatment on the basis of trivial reasons. For example, in one often-discussed case, a Florida urologist posted in his office, "If you voted for Obama... Seek urologic care elsewhere" [41]. This was clearly unethical, for although the physician was not actively harming anybody (thus fulfilling his negative duties), he was failing to help patients who happened to make a political choice (thus neglecting his positive duties).

Of course, positive duties also have limits, even if they are not in conflict with negative duties. This implies that some acts are good, but they are supererogatory actions [42]. *Supererogare* in Latin means to do more than is required. Supererogatory actions are morally commendable and praiseworthy, but they go beyond what is considered morally obligatory or necessary.

Supererogatory actions are typically acts of altruism, self-sacrifice, or extraordinary kindness that exceed the minimum moral standards or duties. These actions are not considered obligatory because they are not required by moral rules, duties, or ethical principles. Instead, they are considered morally exemplary and are often seen as going above and beyond the call of duty.

In the context of medical ethics, various actions would qualify as supererogatory. For example, physicians who voluntarily participate in medical missions to provide care to underserved populations in remote or impoverished areas are performing supererogatory actions. These missions often involve personal sacrifices, such as using vacation time or bearing the financial costs of travel and accommodations. Some physicians also go beyond their professional obligations by providing care to patients who cannot afford it. This may involve offering free or discounted services or helping patients access financial assistance programs or charity care. Likewise, while physicians are expected to provide medical treatment, offering emotional support and comfort to patients and their families in times of distress can be considered a supererogatory action. This goes beyond the technical aspects of care and emphasizes the emotional well-being of patients.

Or consider physicians who engage in medical research to advance knowledge and improve patient care, particularly when they are not obligated to do so. This often involves dedicating extra time and effort to research endeavors. Sometimes patients may even have unusual or unconventional treatment preferences that healthcare providers could accommodate, even if not required to do so. For example, respecting a patient's alternative or complementary treatment choices, when safe and feasible, is a supererogatory action that respects patient autonomy.

But Foot's point is that even if these actions were not supererogatory, failing to fulfill them is not as bad as doing harm. Suppose that for a physician, providing free healthcare to an impoverished patient for free is not supererogatory, but actually ethically required. Nevertheless, the physician who refuses to aid an impoverished patient acts less wrongly than the criminal who steals that patient's money, and as a result, the patient cannot pay for the medical consultation. While the outcome may be the same, in one case a positive duty (aiding the patient by providing medical care) was unfulfilled whereas in the other case a negative duty (not robbing the patient) was unfulfilled.

Foot explained as much with this example: "Most of us allow people to die of starvation in India and Africa, and there is surely something wrong with us that we do; it would be nonsense, however, to pretend that it is only in law that we make the distinction between allowing people in the under-developed countries to die of starvation and sending them poisoned food. There is worked into our moral system a distinction between what we owe people in the form of aid and what we owe them in the way of non-interference" [32].

It is not difficult to appreciate how this line of reasoning can be applied to the ethics of euthanasia. Dr. Kevorkian certainly felt the duty to help his patients, by assisting them in their efforts to be relieved of pain. He had the duty to bring aid. But if in order to bring aid, he had to kill them, this would not be justified. For, he was inflicting an injury on the patients, and the duty not to inflict injury is greater than the duty to bring aid. Many physicians bring aid to their dying patients when they request their treatment to be withdrawn or discontinued. But Foot's ethical stance implies that this is not of the same moral caliber as actively participating in the patients' death, since we are not responsible in the same degree for what we do not do, as for what we do. When a patient dies because a respirator has been disconnected, the physician who disconnects the machine is not participating in the patient's death to the same degree as when a lethal injection is administered. The physician who disconnects the respirator is letting the patient die, but this is fundamentally different than *killing* the patient.

Foot's reasoning implies that euthanasia is closer to the judge who kills an innocent man in order to appease a community, than the physician who prefers to administer the life-saving drug to five patients instead of one. This does not imply that it is never acceptable to kill. The driver is allowed to divert the tram to kill one person, because in so doing, he is avoiding killing five. Both options are his own responsibility, so he must choose the action that minimizes the harm. But that is not the case with the physician who practices euthanasia. The physician is not authorized to kill the patient, because the alternative is the continuation of the patient's pain. The patient's pain is a very bad prospect indeed, but the physician cannot be held responsible for it. The physician has the positive duty to try to alleviate that pain, but the greater negative duty to not cause any harm.

However, this raises the interesting possibility of a physician who is considering practicing euthanasia on a patient who is suffering *as a result* of the physician's previous malpractice. In that case, is the physician ethically authorized to kill the patient, provided the patient requests it? If we assume that the patient's pain is a greater harm than death itself, then the physician would be in a position similar to that of the tram's driver. The physician's dilemma would no longer be between doing and allowing harm, but rather, between choosing the lesser harm.

Most opponents of euthanasia would probably claim that even in such cases, euthanasia is not permissible. Yet, their case would not appeal to the difference between doing and allowing harm, but rather to the claim that death cannot be worse than suffering itself, no matter how intense it may be.

This type of reasoning is in line with the doctrine of the sanctity of life [43]. This doctrine is often associated with religious and moral traditions, particularly within Judaism, Christianity and Islam. Many religious groups hold that life is a divine gift and should not be intentionally taken. The doctrine holds that all human life is inherently sacred and valuable. This doctrine asserts that human life is inviolable and should be protected and preserved under all circumstances, regardless of the individual's age, health, or any other factors. The sanctity of life principle asserts that human life is inviolable, meaning that it should not be intentionally harmed or taken. It opposes euthanasia on the grounds that it violates the inherent sanctity of human life. In its application, it purports to reach all human beings, regardless of their circumstances, characteristics, or abilities.

The doctrine of the sanctity of life is itself subject to various criticisms [44]. Given that this doctrine usually derives from the notion that life is a gift from God and therefore is sacred, it is questionable whether our moral decisions ought to be grounded in religious beliefs. Basing moral and ethical principles on religious beliefs can be exclusionary and may not be appropriate in secular societies that embrace a diversity of religious and non-religious perspectives.

The doctrine also fails to account for nuances and complexities in certain situations. In cases of severe and irreversible suffering or when an individual has a terminal illness, it may be argued that the doctrine prolongs suffering and hinders compassionate end-of-life choices.

Furthermore, if taken to its logical extreme, the doctrine of the sanctity of life may conflict with elementary notions of autonomy. It may limit a person's ability to make decisions about her own life and death, particularly in end-of-life situations or when a person wishes to refuse life-sustaining treatment. Foot's moral reasoning implies that letting die is not as reprehensible as killing, but an overzealous upholding of the doctrine of the sanctity of life may led us to conclude that physicians must not comply with a patient's request to withdraw treatment, since life must be preserved at all costs.

In any case, although perhaps on a popular level much opposition to euthanasia relies on religious notions of the sanctity of life, philosophical debate on this topic has revolved more around the distinction between killing and letting die, which Foot endorsed. Foot used many examples to illustrate her point, but the case of the tram left a marking impression on readers. The most notorious of such readers was Judith Jarvis Thomson, who modified Foot's original tram thought experiment, in order to attempt to prove that, in fact, the distinction between killing and letting die may not be as relevant as at first assumed. In turn, this may require us to rethink the ethics of euthanasia.

## The Challenge to the Killing and Letting Die Distinction

Although Philippa Foot set the foundations of trolleyology, it was Judith Jarvis Thomson who truly set it in motion. Her paper "Killing, Letting Die and the Trolley Problem" had arguably an even greater influence than Foot's [45]. Like Foot, Thomson was interested in seeking an answer to the original question: in what circumstances is it allowed to kill? Like Foot, she resisted raw utilitarianism, and agreed that numbers cannot be the sole criterion in making moral decisions.

Foot had presented the case of the judge who kills an innocent man in order to appease a mob; Thomson adapted that scenario to a situation in medical ethics. She considers the following case: "David is a great transplant surgeon. Five of his patients need new parts-one needs a heart, the others need, respectively, liver, stomach, spleen, and spinal cord-but all are of the same, relatively rare, blood-type. By chance, David learns of a healthy specimen with that very blood-type. David can take the healthy specimen's parts, killing him, and install them in his patients, saving them. Or he can refrain from taking the healthy specimen's parts, letting his patients die" [45].

In recent years, perhaps as a result of conspiracy mongering in the healthcare industry, there have been urban legends about healthy persons being killed in hospitals so as to use their organs to treat a greater number of patients [46]. If such cases exist, they are extremely rare, but the very idea of it happening elicits ethical debate. As in the case of the tram presented by Foot, in this scenario either one dies or five die, yet in this case, the best outcome is for the five to die.

Foot had argued that we can arrive at this conclusion on the basis of the killing and letting die distinction. In her account, killing one is worse than letting five die. But Thomson uses Foot's own tram scenario, and modifies slightly it in order to show that, sometimes, killing one may be preferable than letting five die. Foot had originally presented a tram driver. Thomson preferred to use a trolley to illustrate her point: "Frank is a passenger on a trolley whose driver has just shouted that the trolley's brakes have failed, and who then died of the shock. On the track ahead are five people; the banks are so steep that they will not be able to get off the track in time. The track has a spur leading off to the right, and Frank can turn the trolley onto it. Unfortunately there is one person on the righthand track. Frank can turn the trolley, killing the one; or he can refrain from turning the trolley, letting the five die" [45].

It is important to note that despite its superficial similarity, this case is different from Foot's tram scenario. Here, it is not the trolley driver himself, but someone else, who must make the decision. This implies that Frank did not set the trolley in motion and would therefore not be responsible for the death of the five persons situated on the track. If the trolley is turned, Frank *will* be responsible for the death of the one person. For Frank, then, the dilemma is not between killing five and killing one, but rather, killing one and letting five die.

If Foot is correct, Frank should not divert the trolley. Nobody could accuse him of having killed the five persons. If someone accuses him of having failed to save the five persons, Frank could reply by saying that, in order to do that, he had to kill one person, and his negative duty is more important than his positive duty. This could very well be the same reasoning of the physician who refuses to assist a patient in dying and mounts a defense against those who accuse her of disregarding a patient's pleas and unnecessarily prolonging suffering. Yet, in the case presented by Thomson, it seems that it is at least permissible for Frank to divert the trolley, which implies that killing one is not always worse than letting five die.

The implication of this insight for medical ethics is that sometimes, killing may not be necessarily immoral, even if the alternative is not to kill. The case of Frank would seem to imply that euthanasia may be acceptable, to the extent that there are cases in which it is ethically permissible to kill, even if the agent could simply abstain from doing any action. Frank is permitted to kill one in order to save five who would otherwise be left to die but not actively killed; a physician may kill a patient in order to put an end to suffering, even if otherwise, the patient's suffering would be prolonged, and the patient's death would come from an omission instead of an action.

The distinction between killing and letting die may still be relevant, but Thomson cautions that it cannot be used as an inflexible rule: "the thesis that killing is worse than letting die cannot be used in any simple, mechanical way in order to yield conclusions about abortion, euthanasia, and the distribution of scarce medical resources. The cases have to be looked at individually. If nothing else comes out of the preceding discussion, it may anyway serve as a reminder of this: that there are circumstances in which-even if it is true that killing is worse than letting die-one may choose to kill instead of letting die" [45].

Some philosophers have gone further and have claimed that the killing and letting die distinction is simply useless. The most notorious of these philosophers is James Rachels. Rachels was very interested in the ethics of euthanasia, and posited that refusing to kill may prolong suffering, to the point that it becomes inhumane itself. He envisions a patient with throat cancer who requests the physician to end his life. The doctor agrees, but opts to only apply passive euthanasia, thus withdrawing treatment. Rachels considers this to be a terrible choice: "If one simply withholds treatment, it may take the patient longer to die, and so he may suffer more than he would if more direct action were taken and a lethal injection given. This fact provides strong reason for thinking that, once the initial decision not to prolong his agony has been made, active euthanasia is actually preferable to passive euthanasia, rather than the reverse" [47].

But in Rachels' argument, that is not the main point. The more important point is that, morally speaking, there is no difference between killing and letting die. In order to show why, he presents two scenarios as follows: "In the first, Smith stands to gain a large inheritance if anything should happen to his six-year-old cousin. One evening while the child is taking his bath, Smith sneaks into the bathroom and drowns the child, and then arranges things so that it will look like an accident... In the second, Jones also stands to gain if anything should happen to his six-year-old cousin. Like Smith, Jones sneaks in planning to drown the child in his bath. However, just as he enters the bathroom Jones sees the child slip and hit his head, and fall face down in the water. Jones is delighted; he stands by, ready to push the child's head back under if it is necessary, but it is not necessary. With only a little thrashing about, the child drowns all by himself, "accidentally," as Jones watches and does nothing" [47].

Now, Smith killed the child, whereas Jones "merely" let the child die. That is the only difference between them. Did either man behave better than the other, from a moral point of view? Rachels insists that while Smith kills the cousin and Jones only allows him to die, they are both equally morally reprehensible, as "both men acted from the same motive, personal gain, and both had exactly the same end in view when they acted" [47]. As applied to euthanasia, the implications are clear. If Smith and Jones have moral equivalence, then so do Dr. Kevorkian and any conventional physician who complies with a patient's request to withdraw treatment. Both physicians want the best for the patient, and both have exactly the same end in their actions. The fact that one kills and the other simply lets die is irrelevant. Rachels insists that letting die is itself a type of action, and in this regard, it is morally indistinguishable from killing. As he explains, "one may let a patient die by way of not giving medication, just as one may insult someone by way of not shaking his hand. But for any purpose of moral assessment, it is a type of action nonetheless. The decision to let a patient die is subject to moral appraisal in the same way that a decision to kill him would be subject to moral appraisal: it may be assessed as wise or unwise, compassionate or sadistic, right or wrong" [47].

Other philosophers have followed suit. Michael Tooley presents a case that, in his assessment, further undermines the distinction between killing and letting die: "Imagine a machine containing two children, John and Mary. If one pushes a button, John will be killed, but Mary will emerge unharmed. If one does not push the button, John will emerge unharmed, but Mary will be killed. In the first case one kills John, while in the second case one merely lets Mary die" [48]. As per the killing and letting die distinction, it would be better not to push the button. But Tooley insists that, ultimately, both scenarios are equally bad, and therefore, "the best action, it would seem to me, would be to flip a coin to decide which action to perform, thus giving each person an equal chance of surviving. But if that isn't possible... [it is a] matter of indifference whether one pushes the button or not" [48]. Consequently, if withdrawing treatment and injecting a substance will both result in the patient's death, then there is no relevant different between both alternatives. If injecting the substance will bring a quicker end to the patient's suffering, then it is morally authorized.

Peter Singer argues similarly. In considering the case of an elderly lady with advanced dementia and who has acquired pneumonia, Singer ponders whether there is a significant difference between withholding antibiotic treatment, and administering an injection that would bring about the peaceful death of the patient. Singer arrives at this conclusion: "in both cases, the outcome is the death of the patient. In both cases, the doctor knows that this will be the result and decides what she will do on the basis of this knowledge, because she judges this result to be better than the alternative. In both cases, the doctor must take responsibility for her decision—it would not be correct for the doctor who decided not to provide antibiotics to say that she was not responsible for the patient's death because she did nothing. Doing nothing in this situation is itself a deliberate choice, and one cannot escape responsibility for its consequences" [49].

Although Rachels and Tooley's thought experiments present a challenge, it still seems commonsensical that killing and letting die are not at the same moral level. It seems very counterintuitive that not aiding is equivalent to harming. In fact, most of us refuse to aid almost on a daily basis. We could always give more of our salary to some charity cause, and as a result, some children in an underdeveloped country would be saved from malaria. Indeed, we should give more. But it seems very implausible to argue that not giving to charity in order to save children is the same as killing children. The moral failure of not giving enough is not comparable to the moral failure of killing another human being.

It may be argued that human beings have weak wills, and that explains why most people fail to fulfill their positive duties to the same extent as they fulfill their negative duties. According to this argument, we may have weak wills, but moral demands remain the same, and our duty is to try to meet those demands as much as we can. But that is not a good argument. For, when someone fails to fulfill negative duties (such as not killing), we are very unlikely to say that they are simply weak, but rather, we would say that it is much graver than that. They would not be weak; they would be morally depraved.

Frances Kamm makes the case as follows: "when somebody says, 'My theory implies that you should be giving $1000 to save someone's life and that failing to do so is just as bad as killing someone' and he also says, 'I don't give the $1000 because I'm weak!,' then I can't believe he really thinks he has that obligation to aid and that his not aiding is equivalent to killing. Imagine him saying, 'I just killed someone for $1000 because I'm weak.' Give me a break! This is ridiculous. Either there is something wrong with that theory, or there is something wrong with its proponents" [50].

Furthermore, Richard Trammell argues that the negative duty of not killing has an element of dischargeability that the positive duty of giving to charity lacks. We can discharge on others the duty not to kill anyone, but we cannot discharge on other the duty to save the children from starvation. Collapsing the distinction between doing and allowing harm demands too much from us. As Trammell phrases it, "denial of the distinction between negative and positive duties leads straight to an ethic so strenuous that it might give pause even to a philosophical John the Baptist" [51]. Not only is this ethos unrealistic, but it is also dangerous. For, an ascetic could give away all his money to stop children from starving in a remote country, and when the ascetic finds himself with no money but learns that there are still remaining children to be fed, he would steal from others in order to fulfill his duty to prevent children from starving. Since the duty not to steal is on the same level as the duty to feed children, so he could argue, he may very well be justified in stealing, inasmuch as the victims of his robbery would not starve as a result, whereas his beneficiaries would starve if he does not steal.

We can appeal to other trolley scenarios themselves in order to conclude that there is indeed a relevant distinction between doing and allowing harm. For example, Frances Kamm presents the case of a trolley headed towards five people, and it can be diverted towards another track, also with five people [52]. Should a bystander divert the trolley? Tooley would suggest that we should be indifferent towards which of the two options is chosen. But Kamm insists that it would be better for a bystander *not* to divert the trolley. It should not, as in Tooley's case, be left to the flipping of a coin. Indeed, the outcome with either alternative will be the same, but there is something about *not* causing the harm that influences our decision. In this case, although the outcome is the same, letting die is better than killing.

Although Thomson modified the trolley case so as to show that in some instances, killing one may be preferable to letting five die, she nevertheless acknowledges that in many other cases, the distinction between doing and allowing harm is still relevant. Thomson presents the following scenarios: "Alfrieda knows that if she cuts off Alfred's head he will die, and, wanting him to die, cuts it off; Bertha knows that if she punches Bert in the nose he will die-Bert is in peculiar physical condition-and, wanting him to die, punches him in the nose. But what Bertha does is surely every bit as bad as what Alfrieda does. So cutting off a man's head isn't worse than punching a man in the nose" [45]. Thomson argues that this conclusion is absurd. Yes, both Alfrieda and Bertha have the intention of killing a man, and both of their actions result in deaths. But it is not the case that beheading someone is as bad as punching someone in the nose. There are different degrees of moral viciousness in actions, even with equivalence of intentions and results. And if those degrees exist, then doing harm is worse than allowing harm, even if ultimately, the consequences are the same.

Yet, the challenge remains of how to refute Rachels' claim that Jones and Smith are morally indistinguishable. Rachels is confident that Jones and Smith are equally condemnable. But perhaps that is not altogether accurate. If so, Jones is deeply immoral for not having rescued the cousin out of pure greed; but Smith is slightly more immoral for having actually killed the cousin. In a case such as this one, our intuitions may not be sufficiently capable of figuring out distinctions. The depravity of both characters is so great that we come to think that they are equivalent, when in fact they are not. There is a confounding factor that intuitively obfuscates the distinction, but the distinction is nevertheless real. Richard Trammell sensibly makes the point as follows: "The fact that one cannot distinguish the taste of two wines when both are mixed with green persimmon juice, does not imply that there is no distinction between the wine" [51]. Green persimmon juice obfuscates the distinction between wines, in the same way that greed obfuscates the distinction between doing and allowing harm. That does not imply that the distinction is illusory.

If we find some moral element in Smith's case that is lacking in Jones' case, we ought to uphold the killing and letting die distinction. Frances Kamm believes one such element pertains to restitution [53]. Suppose we could bring back the child to life if we kill someone. Kamm claims that in this scenario, we may kill Smith, but not Jones. As morally depraved as he was, Jones did not kill the child, and therefore, it is not right to kill him to bring back the child to life. The same cannot be said of Smith. And given this difference in the approach to restitution, there does seem to be a relevant distinction between doing and allowing harm.

In any case, for the sake of argument, we may assume that Jones and Smith are morally equivalent in their actions. But in other scenarios, such as euthanasia, the difference between killing and letting die is still sustained. In some cases, although the distinction between killing and letting die holds, Smith and Jones may be morally equivalent for other reasons, and not because killing and letting die are the same. Smith and Jones may be morally equivalent simply because they are both extremely greedy.

To have a cousin die (regardless of whether it is by actively drowning him or merely by letting him drown) in order to inherit some money, is morally wrong. Therefore, it does not matter how this outcome is brought about, since in this case, both killing and letting die are wrong. But in other contexts, the distinction is relevant. Rachels seemed to think that finding one counterexample is enough to undermine the relevance of the distinction between killing and letting die. Yet, that is not necessarily the case. Rachels found one type of situation in which, admittedly, the difference between killing and letting die seems irrelevant. Seeking a young cousin's death out of pure greed is so bad that, indeed, it matters little how the young cousin's death is brought about. But when greed is not involved, the difference is significant. Frances Kamm explains that "it may be that in some equalized contexts, a harming and a not-aiding will be judged as being morally equivalent, yet in other equalized contexts, they will not be" [53].

Consider two cases of a mountain rescuer presented by Fionna Woollard: "In the first case, you are driving Alastair and Bryan to the hospital for life-saving treatment. You see that Charlie is trapped on the hillside. A boulder is rolling towards him and he will be crushed to death by it unless you save him. You could save him, but it would delay you so that it would be too late to save Alastair and Bryan. You drive on. In the second case, the boulder is blocking the route to the hospital. The only way to get to the hospital is to push the boulder towards Charlie, who is trapped on the hillside. You push the boulder" [29]. There is no greed involved here; instead, it is all about pure altruism. As a mountain rescuer, you want to save a greater number of lives (Alastair and Bryan), and in both cases, Charlie will die. But in the first case, you will merely let Charlie die, whereas in the second case, you will kill Charlie. Is there a difference between the two? It certainly seems so. The first case is morally preferred. Although the outcome will be the same, it is better to achieve it by letting die instead of killing.

Even assuming that Smith and Jones are morally equivalent, that does not imply that the distinction between killing and letting die is irrelevant. The important thing may be whether it is harder to justify doing harm than merely allowing it. Consider this argument presented by Warren Quinn: "Your right of privacy that the police not enter your home without permission, for example, is more easily defeated than your right that I, an ordinary citizen, not do so. But it seems morally no better, and perhaps even worse, for the police to violate this right than for me to" [54]. In this case, both the police and an ordinary citizen do wrong by entering someone's house. But it is much harder to justify if the police do it. Consequently, in some cases, killing and letting die may indeed be equivalent, but it is still much harder to justify killing over letting die. That implies that the distinction is indeed relevant.

However, even if the distinction between killing and letting die is relevant, does that entail that euthanasia is morally wrong? Not necessarily. Again, as per Quinn's argument, the relevant aspect is to determine whether it is harder to justify killing than letting die. But that does not imply that killing can never be justified. Passive euthanasia is relatively easy to justify: on the basis of autonomy, it is almost universally accepted that no treatment should be forced on a patient. Active euthanasia is harder to justify, but not impossible. Considerations of compassion may warrant the ethical soundness of active euthanasia. If the patient is requesting an end to her suffering, and it is within the physician's power to provide it, on what grounds can it be refused? Even accepting that killing is worse than letting die, in this case, killing would not be bad.

Although the trolley scenarios I have discussed in this chapter have been relevant to the discussion on the ethics of euthanasia, none of them are sufficiently close to the reality of euthanasia itself. Consequently, whatever intuitions we may have in each of those trolley scenarios, they may not entirely reflect the ethical aspects involved in euthanasia. A much simpler trolley scenario reflecting euthanasia would be as follows: A railway worker has suffered a horrible accident and is being consumed by flames while laying on the tracks; he will likely die in about five minutes, and the burns are now so severe that nobody can save him; he is desperately screaming asking someone to put an end to his misery by killing him. As he screams, a trolley is on its way along the tracks, and will run over the unfortunate worker. A bystander hears the screams and could pull the lever to divert the trolley onto other tracks, thus allowing the worker to live a bit longer, albeit in a horrible, agonizing condition.

Should the trolley be diverted? I posit that no, it should not. The worker is desperately asking someone to kill him, and if the trolley is not diverted, the worker will die and the suffering will mercifully come to an end. The bystander can simply watch as the events unfold, without doing anything, and in that endeavor, suffering will be lessened.

But what if the tracks are reversed? Suppose the worker being consumed in flames is on the diverting track. Should the bystander pull the lever? I posit that, yes, he should. By pulling the lever, the bystander will provide a humane and compassionate option for the worker who is experiencing unbearable suffering. The worker is desperately asking for it, so pulling the lever respects his autonomy, to the extent that it fulfills his wish. Individuals have the right to make decisions about their own lives; respecting a person's autonomy is a fundamental ethical principle.

Is this decision harder to justify than in the first case? Yes, it is. The bystander has to get involved in another person's death. But does that imply that the decision in the first case is justifiable whereas in the second case it is not? No, it does not.

Active euthanasia is harder to justify than passive euthanasia, and this implies that there is indeed an important difference between killing and letting die. But active euthanasia may still be acceptable, for the relevant criterion in order to decide its morality may not necessarily be whether negative duties are more important than positive duties. Trolley scenarios can help us enhance our analytic acumen, but they only provide a provisional guide. As Thomson insisted, reflection on the killing and letting die distinction (and for that matter, most moral principles) cannot be taken as rigid mechanical blueprints about how to proceed morally. Cases still have to be looked at individually, even if trolley scenarios shed light on them.

## The Moral Intricacies of Euthanasia

After having examined the variants of trolley cases that help us clarify our moral intuitions regarding killing and letting die, let us now return to the practice of euthanasia itself in order to arrive at some more robust conclusions concerning its moral status.

Regardless of the way the euthanasia debate may be illustrated by appealing to trolley scenarios, it is also important to consider some arguments that are frequently levelled against euthanasia. Much is made of the concern that, if euthanasia were freely practiced, trust in healthcare providers would be eroded [55, 56].

As per this argument, euthanasia could potentially undermine trust in the medical profession if patients fear that doctors may prioritize economic or societal factors over their best interests. Patients might worry that they will not receive optimal care or that their doctors might suggest euthanasia as a shortcut to dealing with complex medical issues.

Trust concerns also extend to vulnerable populations, such as the elderly, disabled, or mentally ill. If euthanasia were legalized, these groups might feel pressured or coerced into choosing death rather than facing the burden of their medical conditions. It is frequently argued that trust in society's commitment to protect vulnerable individuals could be eroded if euthanasia were seen as an acceptable solution to complex social or economic problems.

There is also the pressing concern that if euthanasia becomes more common, healthcare professionals would neglect their responsibility towards palliative care of those close to death, since they may be hastened to propitiate the patient's death [57, 58]. In such a situation, there's a possibility of healthcare resources being diverted from palliative care services. Euthanasia may emerge as a perceived cost-effective and expedited measure to alleviate suffering, potentially altering cultural perceptions around end-of-life care. This shift might diminish the emphasis on palliative care, favoring instead swift resolutions to suffering. Consequently, healthcare practitioners may show reduced inclination toward aggressive symptom management and holistic patient support. Ethicist Leon Kass raises the concern by asking: "Will doctors be able to care wholeheartedly for patients when it is always possible to think of killing them as a 'therapeutic option'" [59]?

A further worry regarding euthanasia is that it might lead to unintended consequences, and ultimately, society may become desensitized towards grossly immoral procedures. This is a variant of so-called "slippery slope arguments" [60–63]. As per this stance, once a society accepts the practice of euthanasia under certain circumstances, it may gradually expand to include situations that were not originally intended or justified. For example, there may be pressure to extend eligibility criteria of euthanasia to include individuals with chronic illnesses, disabilities, or mental health conditions. This expansion could occur as a result of changing societal attitudes, economic considerations, or advocacy efforts by interest groups.

In marginalized communities, including individuals with disabilities or mental health conditions, there could be an exacerbation of pressure or coercion towards choosing euthanasia, driven by societal stigma, inadequate support systems, or economic adversity. Furthermore, an argument may emerge regarding the normalization of death as a solution to life's adversities by embracing euthanasia, potentially corroding societal norms regarding the sanctity of human life and the necessity of comprehensive palliative care and support for those facing severe illnesses.

While acknowledging the significance of these considerations, there are compelling counterarguments that could sway moral approval towards euthanasia. It is not entirely clear whether the availability of euthanasia would deplete the resources for palliative care [64]. Some individuals confronting terminal illnesses might opt for palliative care to extend their lives, while others might perceive life, even with optimal palliative measures, as lacking adequate quality. The provision of euthanasia does not obviate the requirement for palliative care; rather, it introduces an additional choice for those deeming it appropriate.

Empirical evidence suggests that in jurisdictions where euthanasia is legalized, the availability of palliative care remains unaffected [65]. Although euthanasia is an option, practitioners are always encouraged to make sure patients are aware of possible alternatives. Yet, it is also important to understand that palliative care has limits, and that for some patients, it may not be enough. It would be deeply paternalistic to force palliative measures on patients when, in fact, they prefer to put an end to their suffering once and for all.

Likewise, the extreme scenarios envisioned by those who warn of a slippery slope have not materialized in those territories where euthanasia is readily available, and it is unlikely that they will become commonplace if euthanasia is more widespread. For example, in Oregon, the number of people requesting euthanasia remains low, and the procedure is only used in cases that truly meet the medical profile [66]. Admittedly, euthanasia may be less restricted in countries where it is now legal, but that does not imply that it has fallen along the slippery slope; it may only indicate that people in extreme suffering are now offered better opportunities to put an end to their plight, always complying with the patients' own requests.

In this debate, it is of the utmost importance to consider that patients who seek euthanasia are suffering. In this framework, euthanasia may be considered a compassionate alternative, to the extent that practitioners seek to put an end to such suffering. Individuals facing terminal illnesses or debilitating conditions may endure extreme physical or psychological pain that cannot be adequately alleviated through medical treatment or palliative care. In such cases, euthanasia may be presented as a humane option to end the suffering and provide relief.

Furthermore, we must not lose sight of the fact that prolonging life in the face of unbearable suffering may be ethically questionable, given that it may lead to a prolonged period of distress for the individual and their loved ones. As per this view, euthanasia may be a means to prevent prolonged suffering and allow individuals to die peacefully and on their own terms. To refuse to do so is actually a cruel endeavor.

In fact, euthanasia is routinely practiced on animals undergoing severe suffering, and this elicits little protest [67]. While the nature of animal consciousness is still open to debate, it is safe to assume that there are indeed parallels between the suffering experienced by animals and the suffering endured by humans facing similar circumstances, such as terminal illness, incurable pain, or a severely diminished quality of life. If all such sentient beings deserve compassion, then it would seem incoherent that putting an end to such suffering is only authorized for non-human animals, but not for humans themselves.

In navigating the intricate realm of ethics, there is an imperative for a heightened level of coherence, grappling with the application of principles across diverse scenarios. Should society extend compassion towards animals by embracing euthanasia as a merciful release from suffering, a parallel consideration arises: extending akin compassion to humans confronting analogous predicaments becomes morally compelling.

Beyond the realm of compassion, another ethical cornerstone emerges prominently when dissecting the ethics of euthanasia: autonomy. This principle, intricately intertwined with notions of human dignity and self-governance, stands paramount. Granting patients the agency to exercise autonomy, even in deliberating their continued existence, fosters their active engagement in healthcare decisions, preserving their intrinsic dignity and self-regard.

Autonomy underscores the acknowledgment of the myriad preferences and beliefs individuals harbor concerning end-of-life care. While some may cherish the prospect of euthanasia as a conduit to end their anguish and embrace death with grace, others may opt for aggressive medical interventions or palliative measures. Honoring autonomy necessitates affording individuals the liberty to align their choices with their own ethos and inclinations.

Patients who are undergoing unbearable suffering need compassion the most, precisely because they are at their most vulnerable. In that context, it is only sensible to grant them their wish to decide how to die. Ronald Dworkin makes a meaningful point in asserting that "making someone die in a way that others approve, but he believes a horrifying contradiction of his life, is a devastating, odious form of tyranny" [68]. According to Dworkin's perspective, there exists an inherent entitlement for individuals to shape the trajectory of their existence, encompassing determinations regarding their demise, in alignment with their personal convictions and ideals. The imposition of external judgments or preferences upon an individual's end-of-life decisions transgresses their autonomy and dignity, resulting in a scenario where the individual's essence and integrity are imperiled.

Consider the case of Brittany Maynard, a young woman diagnosed with terminal brain cancer [69]. In 2014, at the age of 29, she gained significant public attention after she publicly announced her decision to move to Oregon in order to access medical aid in dying. Maynard's main argument was that she wanted to preserve her own identity, and she understood that undergoing palliative care would affect her cognitive functioning to the extent that her original psychological identity would hardly be preserved. It would seem quite cruel to refuse her wish to preserve her own self-identity.

Arguments in favor of euthanasia have an important utilitarian dimension. Recall that in the trolley problem variants presented by Foot and Thomson, the people tied to the tracks have no say whatsoever in the decision about whether or not to divert the trolley. In contrast, in the trolley scenario that I have presented above, the person undergoing the horrible burning is desperately requesting others to end their life by diverting the trolley. Good would be maximized if a bystander complies with that person's request.

Prominent utilitarian philosophers have argued along similar lines. For example, Peter Singer insists that euthanasia can be morally justified if it leads to the greatest overall happiness or reduces the greatest amount of suffering. Singer contends that individuals facing terminal illness or debilitating conditions may endure immense physical or psychological pain that cannot be effectively managed through medical treatment or palliative care; in such cases, euthanasia offers a compassionate means of ending suffering and providing relief to the individual.

Certainly, within this framework of thought, the evaluation of the moral permissibility of euthanasia pivots significantly on the notion of quality of life. Individuals grappling with profoundly compromised quality of life, encompassing excruciating pain, erosion of dignity, or an inability to partake in meaningful endeavors, may present compelling justifications for opting for euthanasia.

By ending their lives in such circumstances, individuals can avoid prolonged suffering and maintain a semblance of dignity and control. From a utilitarian perspective, if an individual's suffering outweighs any potential happiness or quality of life they may experience, euthanasia can be considered a morally preferable option. As Singer explains, "voluntary euthanasia occurs only when, to the best of medical knowledge, a person is suffering from an incurable and painful or extremely distressing condition. In these circumstances one cannot say that to choose to die quickly is obviously irrational" [49].

Under a very strict reading of the Hippocratic Oath, one must first do no harm. But as the previous discussion of the trolley scenarios purports to show, there may be exceptional cases in which there is a moral need (if not requirement) to employ some measure of harm in order to achieve greater goods. This also holds in the medical realm. A physician's duty towards patients may sometimes imply a relief of suffering, and in some unfortunate circumstances, that is only achievable by assisting patients in seeking death. In fact, *pace* the critics of euthanasia, this would be the opposite of eroding trust in healthcare professionals. To the extent that a patient knows that a physician will offer help in putting an end to suffering and the physician can be counted on for their empathy, a trust relationship can be built. Certainly, the assurance of not being forsaken by their physicians during their final moments, but rather being supported in achieving the desired end-of-life experience, could indeed foster greater trust among patients.

In the tumultuous landscape of the 1990s, Dr. Kevorkian emerged as a figure of stark division, and even today, his legacy remains ensnared in controversy. This turbulence mirrors the deep-seated schisms within the ongoing cultural battles, a reflection of the intricate and multifaceted nature of the euthanasia discourse. Rooted in ethical, legal, and societal realms, this debate persists, with arguments against euthanasia voicing concerns over healthcare trust erosion, potential neglect of palliative care, and the ominous specter of unintended repercussions. Yet, amid this pattern, there are heavier considerations, underscoring the significance of individual autonomy, compassion, and liberation from excruciating anguish.

I posit that the trajectory toward euthanasia should be charted with respect for autonomy and the alleviation of suffering. Those confronted with terminal illness or insufferable conditions merit the autonomy to determine their own destinies, in alignment with their deeply held beliefs and desires. By heeding the call to honor and uphold individual autonomy, society stands to uphold the pillars of human dignity and empathy in the realm of end-of-life care.

# References

1. Kevorkian J. Capital punishment or capital gain. J Crim Law Crim Police Sci. 1959;50–1.
2. Nieuw AD. Death Med L. 1996;15:319.

3. Hosseini HM. Ethics, the illegality of physician assisted suicide in the United States, and the role and ordeal of Dr. Jack Kevorkian before his death. Rev Eur Stud. 2012;4:203.
4. Euthanasia [Internet]. American Medical Association [cited 2023 Oct 22]. Available from: https://code-medical-ethics.ama-assn.org/ethics-opinions/euthanasia
5. DeCesare M. Death on demand: Jack Kevorkian and the right-to-die movement. Rowman & Littlefield; 2015.
6. Gesang B. Passive and active euthanasia: what is the difference? Med Health Care Philos. 2008;11:175–80.
7. Sanders K, Chaloner C. Voluntary euthanasia: ethical concepts and definitions. Nurs Stand. 2007;21:41–5.
8. Hulett J, Peterson M. Passive Euthanasia Dialogue Nexus. 2014;1:6.
9. Geppert CM, Andrews MR, Druyan ME. Ethical issues in artificial nutrition and hydration: a review. J Parenter Enter Nutr. 2010;34:79–88.
10. Gert B, Culver CM. Distinguishing between active and passive euthanasia. Clin Geriatr Med. 1986;2:29–36.
11. Den Hartogh G. Two kinds of physician-assisted death. Bioethics. 2017;31:666–73.
12. Kuhse H. From intention to consent: learning from experience with euthanasia. In: Physician assisted suicide. Routledge; 2015. p. 252–64.
13. Baksheev AI, Turchina ZE, Mineev V, Maksimov SV, Rakhinsky DV, Aisner LY. Euthanasia in modern society: the topicality, practicability, and medical aspect of the problem. J Pharm Sci Res. 2018;10:1360–3.
14. Rotzoll M, Fuchs P, Richter P, Hohendorf G. Nazi action T4 euthanasia programme: historical research, individual life stories and the culture of remembrance. Nervenarzt. 2010;81:1326–32.
15. Silvestri E. Lebensunwertes Leben: roots and memory of Aktion T4. Conatus-J Philos. 2019;4:65–82.
16. Grodin MA, Miller EL, Kelly JI. The Nazi physicians as leaders in eugenics and "euthanasia": lessons for today. Am J Public Health. 2018;108:53–7.
17. Friedlander H. The T4 killers. The holocaust and history: the known, the unknown, the disputed, and the reexamined; 1998. p. 243–51.
18. Rotzoll M, Richter P, Fuchs P, Hinz-Wessels A, Topp S, Hohendorf G. The first national socialist extermination crime: the T4 program and its victims. Int J Ment Health. 2006;35:17–29.
19. Hinman LM. Euthanasia: the moral landscape. In: Why we kill. Routledge; 2020. p. 124–39.
20. Md Pauzi SF, Omar N. Euthanasia-A comparative study from legal perspective. 2005.
21. Dowbiggin I. From Sander to Schiavo: morality, partisan politics, and America's culture war over euthanasia, 1950–2010. J Policy History. 2013;25:12–41.
22. Racine E, Karczewska M, Seidler M, Amaram R, Illes J. How the public responded to the Schiavo controversy: evidence from letters to editors. J Med Ethics. 2010;36:571–3.
23. Steinbock B, Menzel PT. Bioethics: what everyone needs to know®. Oxford University Press; 2023.
24. Häyry H. Bioethics and political ideology: the case of active voluntary euthanasia. Bioethics. 1997;11:271–6.
25. Cohen J, Van Landeghem P, Carpentier N, Deliens L. Public acceptance of euthanasia in Europe: a survey study in 47 countries. Int J Public Health. 2014;59:143–56.
26. Halman L, Van Ingen E. Secularization and changing moral views: European trends in church attendance and views on homosexuality, divorce, abortion, and euthanasia. Eur Sociol Rev. 2015;31:616–27.
27. Verbakel E, Jaspers E. A comparative study on permissiveness toward euthanasia: religiosity, slippery slope, autonomy, and death with dignity. Public Opin Q. 2010;74:109–39.
28. Lewis P. Rights discourse and assisted suicide. Am J Law Med. 2001;27:45–99.
29. Woollard F. The doctrine of doing and allowing II: the moral relevance of the doing/allowing distinction. Philos Compass. 2012;7:459–69.
30. Smith CM. Origin and uses of primum non nocere—above all, do no harm! J Clin Pharmacol. 2005;45:371–7.

31. Woien S. Life, death, and harm: staying within the boundaries of nonmaleficence. Am J Bioeth. 2008;8:31–2.
32. Foot P. The problem of abortion and the doctrine of the double effect. Appl Ethics: Crit Concepts Philos. 2002;2:187.
33. Hart HLA. Punishment and responsibility: essays in the philosophy of law. Oxford University Press; 2008.
34. Bentham J. A fragment on government; or, a comment on the commentaries. 2. W. Pickering; 1823.
35. Ellenberg SS, Braun MM. Monitoring the safety of vaccines: assessing the risks. Drug Saf. 2002;25:145–52.
36. Miller ER, Moro PL, Cano M, Shimabukuro TT. Deaths following vaccination: what does the evidence show? Vaccine. 2015;33:3288–92.
37. Anscombe G. Who is wronged? Philippa foot on double effect. In: Geach M, Gormally L editors. Human Life, Action and Ethics; 1967. p. 249–51.
38. Domres B, Koch M, Manger A, Becker HD. Ethics and triage. Prehosp Disaster Med. 2001;16:53–8.
39. Berlin I. Four essays on liberty. Oxford University Press; 1969.
40. Beauchamp TL. Promise of the beneficence model for medical ethics. J Contemp Health L Pol'y. 1990;6:145.
41. Florida Doctor Tells Obama Supporters to "Go Elsewhere" for Care. Is that Ethical? [Internet]. ABC News. 2010 [cited 2023 Oct 23]. Available from: https://abcnews.go.com/WN/florida-doctor-tells-obama-supporters-care/story?id=10268425.
42. Stanlick NA. The nature and value of supererogatory actions. J Soc Philos. 1999;30:209–22.
43. Rakowski E. The sanctity of human life. Yale LJ. 1993;103:2049.
44. Keenan JF. The concept of sanctity of life and its use in contemporary bioethical discussion. In: Sanctity of life and human dignity. Springer; 1996. p. 1–18.
45. Thomson JJ. Killing, letting die, and the trolley problem. In: death, dying and the ending of life, vol. I and II. Routledge; 2019. p. V2_17-V2_30.
46. Campion-Vincent V. Organ theft narratives as medical and social critique. J Folklore Res. 2002;33–50.
47. Rachels J. Active and passive euthanasia. In: Death, dying and the ending of life, vol. I and II. Routledge; 2019. p. V2_5-V2_7.
48. Tooley M. An irrelevant consideration: killing versus letting die. Killing Letting Die. 1980;2:103–11.
49. Singer P. Practical ethics. Cambridge: Cambridge University Press; 2011.
50. Voorhoeve A. Conversations on ethics. Oxford University Press; 2009.
51. Trammell RL. Saving life and taking life. J Philos. 1975;72:131–7.
52. Kamm F. Parfit on the irrelevance of deontological distinctions. In: Oxford studies in normative ethics, vol. 10. Oxford University Press; 2020. p. 9–31.
53. Kamm FM. Intricate ethics: rights, responsibilities, and permissable harm. Oxford University Press; 2008.
54. Quinn WS. Actions, intentions, and consequences: the doctrine of doing and allowing. Philos Rev. 1989;98:287–312.
55. Pellegrino ED. Doctors must not kill. In: Death, dying and the ending of life, vol. I and II. Routledge; 2019. p. V2_257-V2_264.
56. Hall M, Trachtenberg F, Dugan E. The impact on patient trust of legalising physician aid in dying. J Med Ethics. 2005;31:693–7.
57. Willard C. Killing and caring: is euthanasia incompatible with care? Eur J Cancer Care. 1997;6:40–4.
58. Janssens MJPA. Palliative care: concepts and ethics. Nijmegen: Nijmegen University Press; 2001.
59. O'Malley S. The slippery slope of assisted suicide [Internet]. 2022. Available from: https://www.thebostonpilot.com/article.php?ID=15219.

60. Ryan CJ. Pulling up the runaway: the effect of new evidence on euthanasia's slippery slope. J Med Ethics. 1998;24:341–4.
61. Gillon R. Euthanasia in The Netherlands–down the slippery slope? J Med Ethics. 1999;25:3.
62. Materstvedt LJ. The Euthanasia debate palliative care on the'slippery slope'towards euthanasia? Palliat Med. 2003;17:387–92.
63. Lerner BH, Caplan AL. Euthanasia in Belgium and the Netherlands: on a slippery slope? JAMA Intern Med. 2015;175:1640–1.
64. Benatar D. A legal right to die: responding to slippery slope and abuse arguments. Curr Oncol. 2011;18:206–7.
65. Gerson SM, Koksvik GH, Richards N, Materstvedt LJ, Clark D. Assisted dying and palliative care in three jurisdictions: Flanders, Oregon, and Quebec. Ann Palliative Med. 2021;10:3528–39.
66. Oregon Death with Dignity Act [Internet]. Oregon Health Authority. 2020. Available from: chrome-extension://efaidnbmnnnibpcajpcglclefindmkaj/, https://www.oregon.gov/oha/PH/PROVIDERPARTNERRESOURCES/EVALUATIONRESEARCH/DEATHWITHDIGNITYACT/Documents/year23.pdf.
67. Kuře J. Euthanasia: The "Good Death" Controversy in Humans and Animals. BoD–Books on Demand; 2011.
68. Dworkin R. Life's dominion: an argument about abortion, euthanasia, and individual freedom. Vintage; 2011.
69. Sandström J. "I will not die that way. Why should I be forced to?": Brittany Maynard's story in the campaign for assisted dying, a narrative perspective. 2019;

References

# Chapter 2
# Abortion

**Abstract** This chapter introduces the history of the *Roe v Wade* decision and its aftermath, so as to discuss the ethics of abortion. One particularly disturbing phenomenon in recent years has been the bombing of abortion clinics, yet through the use of a trolley scenario, I posit that it is not coherent to consider abortion a form of murder and at the same time condemn the bombing of abortion clinics. Furthermore, by considering various trolley scenarios—and other thought experiments—originally formulated by Judith Jarvis Thomson, I discuss the extent to which abortion may be considered a legitimate form of self-defense. While these arguments do not necessarily hinge upon the personhood status of fetuses, this chapter also discusses some of the arguments for and against the idea that embryos and fetuses can be considered persons with moral rights.

In the history of the culture wars, perhaps more divisive than Dr. Jack Kevorkian was Norma McCorvey. The name probably will be unfamiliar to most readers, but certainly her pseudonym "Jane Roe" evokes deep divisions and debates in contemporary society.

In 1969, McCorvey gave birth to a girl. She struggled with motherhood, and McCorvey's own mother took custody of the child. The child was given up for adoption even when McCorvey did not approve of it. In 1969, at the age of twenty-one, McCorvey found herself pregnant with her third child and a serious addiction problem.

She desired to have an abortion, but living in Texas, she had no access to the procedure, as abortion was illegal in that state. At the time, abortion laws in the United States varied widely by state. Many states criminalized or heavily restricted abortion. Abortion rights advocates saw these laws as infringing upon women's reproductive freedom, while opponents argued for the protection of fetal life and the preservation of traditional moral values [1].

McCorvey attempted abortion via illegal means, to no effect. Her friends then persuaded her to seek legal counsel so as to challenge the illegality of abortion. She was referred to Linda Coffee and Sarah Weddington, two young lawyers campaigning for the legalization of abortion.

G. Andrade, *Trolleyology in Medicine*, SpringerBriefs in Ethics,
https://doi.org/10.1007/978-3-031-72806-8_2

In these legal procedures, McCorvey took the pseudonym "Jane Doe." Coffee and Weddington filed a suit against Henry Wade, the district attorney of Dallas County, where McCorvey resided—hence the name of the famous trial, *Roe v Wade*. The case made its way through the legal system, eventually reaching the United States Supreme Court. The central argument revolved around whether a woman had a right to control her body (and by extension, to terminate her pregnancy) on account of rights to privacy [2].

The case garnered extensive media attention and legal commentary, and finally, in January 1973, the Supreme Court handed down a decision dictating that a woman's right to privacy extended to her decision to have an abortion. This right, the Court determined, must be balanced against the State's interest in regulating abortions to protect maternal health and fetal life. The Court established that abortion would only be allowed within the first ninety days of pregnancy [3].

The Supreme Court decision soon became a landmark event in American legal history, with far-reaching implications. The case was a huge stimulus for the reproductive rights movement, as it provided a legal foundation for advocating women's right to control their own bodies and make decisions about their reproductive health. The decision energized activists who had long fought for access to safe and legal abortion, leading to increased visibility and advocacy for reproductive rights issues [4].

For many supporters of women's rights, the *Roe v. Wade* case represented a significant milestone in the struggle for gender equality and autonomy. The ability to control their reproductive choices empowered women to pursue education, careers, and personal goals without the fear of unwanted pregnancy. Access to safe and legal abortion was seen as essential to women's ability to participate fully in society and exercise their fundamental rights.

But unsurprisingly, the case also had a deep polarizing effect. The issue of abortion became deeply divisive, with individuals and groups on both sides of the debate fiercely advocating for their positions. Whereas in the preceding decades liberals and conservatives focused on other issues, abortion became a defining topic in American politics, shaping electoral campaigns, party platforms, and judicial appointments.

The *Roe v. Wade* decision mobilized activists on both sides of the abortion debate. Anti-abortion groups, often aligned with religious organizations, organized grassroots campaigns, protests, and lobbying efforts to restrict abortion rights. Pro-choice advocates, including women's rights organizations and reproductive health advocates, similarly mobilized to defend and expand access to abortion services. This activism intensified the polarization by amplifying competing voices and narratives [5].

*Roe v. Wade* has consistently divided public opinion. Although support of abortion has fluctuated at different times, for the most part, in public opinion there is roughly an equal split between those who support abortion rights and those who oppose them [6]. This polarization is reflected in public discourse, media coverage, and cultural representations of abortion, which often frame the issue in terms of conflicting values and ideologies—a major scenario of confrontation in the culture wars.

Ironically, McCorvey's life had a dramatic turnabout after the trial [7]. By the 1990s, she had engaged with anti-abortion activists, and began to develop an ideological opposition to abortion. She then embraced an active life as a Christian, and her faith became central to her identity and worldview, shaping her moral values and guiding her activism against abortion.

McCorvey's personal story and conversion experience provided a powerful narrative for the pro-life movement. She remained actively involved in legal battles and advocacy efforts aimed at challenging abortion rights and promoting anti-abortion legislation. The fact that she had been the original Jane Roe was seized upon by anti-abortion activists, who could now claim that the very same plaintiff in the landmark case had a change of views. This transformation left a lasting impact on the abortion rights debate in the United States. Her story challenged conventional narratives about abortion and offered a compelling testimonial for those who opposed abortion on moral grounds.

Yet, by the time McCorvey had reverted her original stance, the reproductive rights movement was already in full swing, and this debate continues today. As it happens, abortion is a central issue in medical ethics, and variants of trolley scenarios have been frequently used in order to argue for both sides of the debate. This becomes quite important in considering the ethics of self-defense, as trolley scenarios can help us clarify our intuitions about the limits of self-defense, and in turn, that can guide our moral reasoning towards the issue of abortion.

## Self-defense and the Bombing of Abortion Clinics

Opposition to abortion stems from many fronts, but perhaps none more so than the Catholic Church. The doctrinal stance of the Church is very clear. As it is expressed officially in article 2270 of the Catechism, "human life must be respected and protected absolutely from the moment of conception. From the first moment of his existence, a human being must be recognized as having the rights of a person—among which is the inviolable right of every innocent being to life" [8]. Likewise, article 2272 stipulates that "formal cooperation in an abortion constitutes a grave offense. The Church attaches the canonical penalty of excommunication to this crime against human life" [8]. In article 2274 the Catechism also makes no qualms about the ontological status of the embryo: "since it must be treated from conception as a person, the embryo must be defended in its integrity, cared for, and healed, as far as possible, like any other human being" [8].

However, some scholars have asserted that in previous epochs the Church's doctrine on abortion was not as intransigent as it is today [9–13]. It is true that throughout its history, the Catholic Church has consistently upheld the sanctity of human life. Early Christian writings, such as the Didache and the Letter of Barnabas, explicitly condemned abortion [14]. Early Church fathers like Tertullian, Athenagoras, and Jerome spoke out against abortion, considering it a grave sin [15].

Nevertheless, the Church did not always have a definitive stance on the moral status of embryos. Some authors, such as Gregory of Nyssa and Maximus the Confessor, asserted that human life commenced at conception [16]. In contrast, figures like Lactantius suggested that the soul was "infused" into the body forty days after conception [17]. As per the account of historian John Riddle, staunch Catholic opposition to abortion only began in the 19th Century; prior to that, many Catholic authors—not all—considered licit to end the embryo's life before quickening [18, 19].

Quickening refers to the moment when a pregnant woman first perceives fetal movement in her womb. Historically, quickening was significant because it was believed to mark the point at which the fetus became animated, indicating the presence of a living being. In many cultures and legal systems, quickening was considered a crucial milestone in the development of the fetus and often influenced laws and religious beliefs regarding abortion [20].

Before the advent of modern medical technology, quickening served as a practical and legal distinction regarding the permissibility of abortion. However, with advancements in our understanding of embryology and prenatal development, the concept of quickening has lost much of its significance in both medical and legal contexts. Modern science has demonstrated that fetal movement is a natural part of prenatal development and does not necessarily signify the presence of a fully formed human being with consciousness or personhood.

Perhaps the one philosopher and theologian the Catholic intellectual tradition holds in greatest esteem is Thomas Aquinas. Yet, Aquinas' views on abortion are not identical to the Church's current stance. On the one hand, Aquinas considered abortion to be a grave sin because it violates the natural inclination toward self-preservation and the preservation of innocent human life. On the other hand, Aquinas seemed to believe that the embryo received the soul, not immediately upon conception, but rather, 40 (for males) or 80 (for females) days after [21].

It is important to emphasize that Aquinas never endorsed the morality of abortion, but his views about when the embryo becomes a person are at odds with current Catholic teaching, and this has prompted people on the pro-choice side of the debate to argue that opposition to abortion has not been as stringent as traditionally thought, and consequently, Catholics themselves may reconsider their position on an issue that has been somewhat fluid [13].

Aquinas did not dedicate much attention to either abortion or ensoulment. In contrast, the topic of self-defense was one of his major interests. He embraced the concept of natural law, which holds that moral principles are inherent in the nature of human beings and the world. According to Aquinas, self-preservation is a fundamental instinct deeply ingrained in human nature. Therefore, individuals have a natural right to defend themselves against unjust aggression and harm. In his words, "nothing hinders one act from having two effects, only one of which is intended, while the other is beside the intention. ... Accordingly, the act of self-defense may have two effects: one, the saving of one's life; the other, the slaying of the aggressor" [22]. In self-defense, one seeks to preserve one's life; the aggressor may be killed, but that is not the intention of the self-defense act, albeit it may be foreseeable.

Aquinas categorized self-defense as a form of justifiable action. He argued that individuals have a moral right to use proportionate force to repel an unjust aggressor and protect themselves or others from harm. However, he emphasized that self-defense must be guided by the virtues of prudence, temperance, and justice, rather than driven by vengeance or malice [23].

Taking inspiration from Aquinas, there has been a strong philosophical tradition—both religious and secular—of Just War theory. This normative theory stipulates certain conditions that must be met before the initiation of armed conflict. The first condition is having a just cause, which involves responding to harm inflicted. Secondly, right intention is crucial, to the extent that it is not morally licit to wage war with malicious intentions even if the cause is justifiable. The third element is the principle of last resort, emphasizing the preference for non-violent solutions before resorting to armed conflict. Lastly, the requirement of proportionality dictates that the response to aggression must be proportional to the original offense, ensuring that the force used aligns with the objectives of the conflict.

It is also important to note that, when engaging in warfare, it is essential to ensure that armed actions are directed only towards combatants, as emphasized by the principle of discrimination. This principle dictates that efforts should be made to distinguish between legitimate and illegitimate targets to minimize harm to non-combatants. Additionally, it is crucial to assess the potential military advantages of an attack against the possible harm to civilians and civilian infrastructure. If the harm inflicted upon civilians outweighs the military benefits gained from the attack, the action would be deemed disproportionate and contrary to ethical standards.

Seeing through the lens of proponents of the pro-life movement, the argument surfaces that embryos hold the status of persons, thus framing abortion as the intentional end of a human life. However, delving into this perspective beckons a critical reassessment of how we define personhood when it comes to embryos. The assertion that abortion equates to murder, a staunch stance upheld by anti-abortion entities, leads us down a disquieting path of implications regarding the scale and gravity of the act. Analogously, contemplating abortion as a form of genocide due to the sheer volume of abortions performed each year draws unsettling parallels with past genocidal events in history. In the year 2017 alone, the United States documented a total of 612,719 abortions, [24] a figure remarkably close to the toll seen in historical genocides such as those witnessed in Armenia and Rwanda.

While the yearly rate of abortions in the U.S. remains lower than the catastrophic death toll of events like the Holocaust, considering the cumulative impact of numerous abortions over time reveals a harrowing reality of lives lost. Estimates indicate that the collective death toll attributed to abortions significantly surpasses the tragedies of the Holocaust, amounting to an alarming figure of around 60 million lives extinguished.

Indeed, some religious leaders have had no qualms in saying that abortion is a form of genocide. For example, in his 2005 book *Memory and Identity*, Pope John Paul II stated that abortion and the Holocaust had many similarities. Commenting on Nazis' rise to power, John Paul II added that "we must question certain legislative choices made by the parliaments of today's democratic regimes. The most immediate example concerns abortion laws" [25]. Noted anti-abortion activist Michael Bray likewise insists that "Americans live in a situation comparable to Nazi Germany" [26].

Let us contemplate the hypothesis that if embryos are deemed persons, then abortion clinics are, in essence, perpetrating genocide by ending millions of lives each year. Given this troubling perspective, the ethical dilemma arises: how should society respond morally to what is perceived as genocide? Reflecting on historical injustices like the Holocaust, it is commonly acknowledged that the Jewish population had a rightful basis for resistance. The uprising in the Warsaw ghetto serves as a powerful illustration of defiance against unbearable conditions that no reasonable person would denounce.

Stephen Kershnar envisions the following scenario: "A Nazi worker drives his truck to his job at the death camp, Treblinka. His job is to drop Zyklon B into the shower-like rooms that are used to kill Jews. A Jewish resistance group kills the worker with an anti-tank round when he is a mile away from the camp. They do so in order to save Jewish lives. Under German law, assassinating death camp workers is illegal and punishable by death" [27]. Most people would agree that, on the basis of self-defense and as per the tenets of Just War theory, the Jewish resistance group is authorized to do so, even if it is illegal under German law.

Consider now this trolley scenario: a trolley is conducted by a very malicious driver who deliberately switches tracks in order to run over and kill one thousand people who are tied to that track. A bystander can pull a lever, this will destroy the trolley before running over the thousand people tied to the tracks, and its driver will die. Is it morally right for the bystander to pull the lever?

I posit that, yes, the bystander is at least allowed to do so. This would not be self-defense, but rather as Judith Jarvis Thomson phrases it, "other-defense of more than one" [28]. Surely the bystander is not being threatened by the driver, but the fact is that the driver is an aggressor, and in the same manner that the victims would be entitled to defend themselves against the aggressor, if it is in the bystander's realm of possibility to save the victims, then the bystander should do it, even if it brings about the aggressor's death. As Thomson explains, it is "very plausible to suppose that the permissibility of X's killing Y in self-defense goes hand in hand with the permissibility of Z's killing Y in defense of X, and that both phenomena have a common source" [28].

There is a sense of urgency in this trolley scenario. In other circumstances, the bystander could try to reason with the malicious driver. But there is simply no time, and the urgency requires drastic action. Consequently, the bystander ought to pull the lever. Likewise, perhaps at first some people could have tried to reason with the Nazis, or they could have resorted to non-violent resistance. But given that all of that proved futile and that the number of victims in the Holocaust increased by the day, members of the Jewish resistance were entitled to some violent action targeting the Nazis. That would have been perfectly in line with the tenets of Just War theory and it would have been a legitimate act of self-defense.

Now, let us establish an analogy with abortion clinics. If the genocide is indeed taking place—given that embryos are persons, and millions of embryos are killed every day—then very much as the Jewish resistance group or the bystander pulling the lever to explode the oncoming trolley, it is morally acceptable to use violence in order to attempt to stop the aggressors. In fact, this is what some extremist groups have been doing in the United States by bombing abortion clinics ever since the *Roe v. Wade* decision.

The overwhelming majority of organizations opposing abortion—and even those who deem abortion a form of genocide— disapprove of bombing abortion clinics. For groups like Pro-Lifers Against Clinic Violence and the National Coalition for Life and Peace have issued sentiments, emphasizing that resorting to violence is unjustifiable and falls outside the realm of legitimate activism. The concerns raised by these anti-abortion organizations regarding violent actions are valid, as such behavior rightfully constitutes a crime and should find no support or justification within the anti-abortion movement.

Yet, this stance leads to a paradox. Those advocating for the bombing of abortion clinics could argue that such actions align with principles of self-defense. From this perspective, abortion is perceived as an ongoing and deliberate act of harm. Particularly within countries like the United States, where abortion is not only legalized but also regulated by governmental bodies, the practice can be seen as a systematic form of aggression authorized by the state. The prevalence of abortion procedures carried out in recent decades, both in the U.S. and worldwide, underscores the moral grounds for resisting what is perceived as a constant and institutionally sanctioned form of aggression.

Likewise, in bombing abortion clinics, surely the intention is right—i.e., saving millions of fetuses, in the same manner that the bystander pulling the lever would have the right intention: saving the thousand people tied to the track. If somehow the trolley explodes but the evil trolley driver survives, surely the bystander pulling the lever would not be saddened. The ultimate goal is to save the victims, not to gratuitously kill the aggressors.

Similarly, those involved in the anti-abortion movement are largely motivated by a desire to prevent abortions rather than deriving pleasure from harm inflicted upon abortion providers. This even includes those who support the bombing of clinics. For example, Michael Bray has argued that "unborn children" ought to be saved by "destroying the facilities that they are regularly killed in, or taking the life of one who is murdering them" [29]. In his view, this is a justifiable act because it is not done in the spirit of revenge or to play the part of both judge and executioner, but rather, to save lives. In Bray's words, "there is a difference between taking a retired abortionist and executing him, and killing a practicing abortionist who is regularly killing babies" [29]. Ending the life of the retired abortionist serves no moral justification, while targeting the practicing abortionist serves a defensive purpose by preventing further abortions performed by the doctor subjected to the bombing.

When exploring the ethical considerations surrounding self-defense, it becomes imperative to uphold a principle known as the last resort. Applying this concept to the trolley dilemma, initial attempts may involve efforts to reason with the trolley driver to halt its course. However, once it becomes evident that persuasion is futile and the trolley is dangerously close to calamity, the final recourse is to act decisively by pulling the lever to trigger the trolley's detonation.

Drawing a parallel analogy towards the bombing of abortion clinics, a similar line of reasoning emerges. Admittedly, this standard may seemingly conflict with justifications for violent actions within the anti-abortion movement. Initially, individuals may choose to pursue legal avenues to challenge the legality of abortion across different jurisdictions. Through political advocacy and lobbying endeavors, the potential for legislative changes exists, which could lead to the outlawing of abortion practices, consequently resulting in the closure of clinics and a marked decrease in abortion procedures. Consequently, resorting to violent measures against abortion clinics may not align with the principle of last resort, given that there remains a glimmer of hope for achieving a legal framework where abortion is prohibited.

Yet, while there are indications of possible future developments, it is far from certain that abortion would be illegalized in many countries, and if it does occur, it would likely be a long-term process. Meanwhile, over half a million abortions continue annually solely in the United States. If abortion is deemed equivalent to murder, then waiting for non-violent solutions may not be viable. Despite over 40 years of efforts to criminalize abortion, there has been little success. Therefore, proponents of violent anti-abortion actions may argue that the sheer number of victims justifies their actions, as waiting for peaceful resolutions is impractical.

Proportionality may also be a concern. Sound ethical reasoning would suggest that in responding to aggression with armed action, the response should not exceed the initial offense, aiming for proportionality between force used and objectives pursued. If the use of force results in excessive destruction disproportionate to the objective, then the armed action should not proceed. But again, if abortion is murder and a genocide is currently taking place, then this should not be truly a concern, for the proportionality would be preserved.

If the lever were pulled, the driver would die in the explosion. The number of casualties is minimized, focusing on one individual to save one thousand innocent people tied to the tracks. Similarly, in the targeted bombing of an abortion clinic, casualties are likely to be relatively few, as these are not indiscriminate attacks but rather are focused on abortion facilities. In fact, most violent anti-abortion incidents have resulted in relatively low numbers of casualties [30]. If the attack succeeds, the number of saved fetuses significantly outweighs the casualties from the attack. With abortion providers no longer present and facilities rendered inoperable, a substantial number of fetuses are saved, ensuring that the harm caused by the armed action remains proportional to the good achieved.

Of course, acts of self-defense must also solely target aggressors. But those who bomb clinics also meet this requirement. If abortion is considered equivalent to murder, then both abortion clinics and those who provide abortions (including physicians, nurses, and anyone else working in such facilities) are deemed legitimate targets, as they are directly involved in causing harm. It is crucial to note that these targets must be actively engaged in harmful activities. Remember, Bray argues against targeting retired abortion providers because the objective of the bombings is not solely to cause harm but rather to save fetuses. Killing retired physicians will not contribute to this goal, whereas targeting active physicians who regularly perform abortions will.

However, the bystander may wonder if, upon pulling the lever, the explosion would kill innocent people riding on the trolley, other bystanders, or even worse, some of the thousand people tied to the tracks. In that case, should the lever be pulled? Likewise, it must be acknowledged that in the bombing of abortion clinics, there is always the risk of causing harm to bystanders who are neither culpable nor actively engaged in wrongdoing. Additionally, there is the troubling possibility that some fetuses may be harmed or killed in the process, which appears to contradict the intended purpose entirely.

In acts of self-defense, the killing of bystanders may be a morally contentious issue. Judith Jarvis Thomson considers the following scenario: "A villain has started a trolley toward you... You cannot deflect the trolley at all, you can only fire your antitank gun at it. But there is a bystander standing next to the trolley track, and if you fire your antitank gun, you will blow up the bystander along with the trolley" [28]. Thomson argues that this action would not be morally acceptable. The bystander is not at fault for the deeds of the villain, so why should he pay the price?

As a reply, it may be posited that there are numerical considerations at stake. Thomson herself hints at this: "[an] interesting kind of variant on these cases is what we get when we imagine that what is in question is not self-defense but other-defense, and moreover, not merely other-defense but other-defense of more than one" [28]. When there is only one life to save, it may be morally dubious to pursue an action that kills an innocent bystander. But if one thousand lives are at stake (as in the original trolley scenario we have been discussing), then the death of one bystander may be justified as a side-effect of an action to save one thousand.

Indeed, Thomson acknowledges that in times of war, a pilot on the just side of the war may drop a bomb on the enemy's munition factory, and if as an unintended side-effect some innocent children die, it may still be morally acceptable. She calls that hypothetical pilot a "strategic bomber," and she upholds the morality of his action. She writes: "How does the fact that there is a war on in Strategic Bomber do the moral work of making it permissible for the pilot to proceed? At least partly, I am sure, by virtue of making it the case that the (long-range) stakes are higher than we have been told about in being told about those children in the hospital next door to the munitions factory" [28].

In other words, in the context of just and legitimate wars, unintentionally killing bystanders in self-defense is morally admissible, to the extent that the stakes are much higher than in isolated acts of self-defense. If we embrace this reasoning, then even if some innocent people die, bombing abortion clinics serves a moral purpose. For, in this type of action, the stakes are very high. After all, the bombing of the abortion clinic seeks to stop an alleged genocide, and there can hardly be a situation with higher stakes.

Furthermore, we may appeal to the doctrine of double effect. We shall discuss the doctrine later on in this chapter, but for now, it suffices to say that, as per its tenets, an agent may undertake an action even if they foresee that it will result in both favorable and unfavorable consequences, such as the inadvertent harm to bystanders. Those who place bombs in abortion clinics may indeed anticipate that their actions will lead to adverse effects, such as the loss of innocent lives or even harm to fetuses. However, they also anticipate that their actions will ultimately save numerous fetuses, which is a positive outcome. As long as their actions have a dual effect, they are deemed ethically permissible.

Violent activists against abortion aim solely for the positive outcome. If they had the means to prevent abortions without harming fetuses or bystanders, they would likely opt for it. Their sole intention is to prevent the loss of fetuses, not to mete out punishment to wrongdoers. While it is acknowledged that fetuses and innocent bystanders may perish in these bombings, such actions are still deemed ethically acceptable because the loss of fetuses or bystanders is not a means to the positive outcome of saving more fetuses.

While it is regrettable that ten innocent passengers may die once the trolley explodes, that number is far lower than the one thousand people who would die if the lever were not pulled. Likewise, in bombing abortion clinics one may anticipate that innocent bystanders and fetuses may lose their lives, but that number is expected to be significantly lower than the fetuses saved through such violent actions. Considering the high volume of abortions conducted daily in clinics across the United States and other countries, this becomes particularly relevant.

It is extremely important to note that the argument I have presented is not an endorsement of violence or destructive actions. Instead, it seeks to highlight a moral and logical inconsistency within the anti-abortion movement. By drawing a parallel between the perceived act of murder (abortion) and the extreme response (bombing), the aim is to demonstrate the problematic nature of equating abortion with murder.

Proponents of the anti-abortion stance often argue that abortion is equivalent to taking a human life, thus categorizing it as murder. If this were consistently applied, drastic actions to prevent such "murders"—as Jews resisting the Holocaust—might be seen as morally defensible. However, the vast majority of anti-abortion advocates would condemn violent attacks on clinics and healthcare providers, recognizing that such actions are ethically untenable. This discrepancy suggests that the comparison between abortion and murder is not as straightforward or universally applicable as some might assert.

By exploring this inconsistency, the intent is to challenge the foundational premise of the anti-abortion argument. If bombing clinics is broadly viewed as an unjustifiable and extreme measure, despite the belief that abortion is murder, it calls into question the initial classification of abortion as a murderous act. The hope is to foster a deeper, more nuanced discussion about the ethics surrounding abortion and to encourage anti-abortion supporters to reconsider their position in light of this moral contradiction.

Abortion is not murder because, simply, the embryo is not yet a person. This is of course a very intricate debate, and we will come back to it later on in this chapter. But let us consider another trolley scenario as a provisional hint of the embryo's moral status. A trolley is on its way to run over five embryos preserved in petri dishes; the trolley can be diverted to another track in which one person is tied. Should the driver divert it? If the embryos were persons, then as in Foot's original trolley scenario, the driver should indeed divert the trolley, because the difference is between killing one and killing five. But is that really the case? More empirical work needs to be done in this area, but presumably, most people would agree that the driver should not divert the trolley. This indicates that the dilemma is *not* between killing one and killing five. At most, the dilemma would be between killing five entities with the potential to be persons and killing one person. If indeed most people would choose to not divert the trolley, then that would indicate that, at bottom, they may acknowledge that the embryos are potentially persons, but they still do not outweigh the one person tied to the tracks. Consequently, ontologically speaking, the embryos are still less than persons, for if they were, there would be justification in diverting the trolley, but there is no such justification. If embryos are less than persons, then killing them is not the same as murder, for the crime of murder only applies to persons.

Nevertheless, it seems plausible that at some point in pregnancy, the fetus does become a person. Most countries that have legalized abortion have set the line at ninety days, and indeed, an embryo in a petri dish (as in the trolley scenario) would be before that stage. But let us consider another trolley scenario: this time, the trolley is on its way to kill four women tied to the track, and each of those women are in their ninth month of pregnancy; the driver can divert the trolley towards the other track, where five non-pregnant women are tied. Should the trolley be diverted?

Again, this scenario needs to be tested empirically, but we may anticipate that, as compared to the previous trolley scenario, more people would approve diverting the trolley. In one reckoning (presumably of most people), the dilemma here is between killing eight and killing five. In many jurisdictions throughout the world, killing a woman with an advanced pregnancy would be considered a double homicide if both the woman and the fetus were killed. This legal concept is often referred to as "fetal homicide" [31, 32]. The specific laws regarding fetal homicide vary by jurisdiction, but in many places, killing a pregnant woman resulting in the death of her fetus is treated as a separate offense in addition to the homicide of the woman herself. These laws recognize the fetus as a victim with its own legal rights, distinct from those of the pregnant woman. If we extend this legal reasoning to the trolley scenario, in diverting the trolley, we would be saving four women and four additional persons.

Of course, not every murder of a pregnant woman is considered a fetal homicide. Some jurisdictions may have different legal thresholds for when fetal homicide laws apply based on gestational age. In most cases, laws follow the ninety-day threshold that is established for the legality of abortion.

Interestingly, presumably some ethicists would favor not turning the trolley in the case presented above. In their view, 9-month-old fetuses and even newly born children do not outweigh the moral status of adults. For example, Michael Tooley has discussed infanticide within the context of abortion and the moral status of infants. Tooley argues for a view known as "gradualism," which posits that the moral status of a being increases gradually as it develops certain characteristics, rather than having an all-or-nothing status from conception or birth [33].

Tooley suggests that newborn infants lack certain psychological capacities that are typically associated with personhood, such as self-awareness, rationality, and the ability to form complex desires. Because of this, he argues that killing a newborn infant is not morally equivalent to killing a person with fully developed cognitive capacities. Instead, he contends that it may be morally permissible to end the life of a newborn under certain circumstances, such as severe disability or if the infant's continued existence would cause significant suffering to themselves or others.

Tooley emphasizes the difference between persons and human beings. Fetuses may be human beings, but they are not fully formed persons yet, and therefore, do not have an unqualified right to life. In Tooley's words, "an organism possesses a serious right to life only if it possesses the concept of a self as a continuing subject of experiences and other mental states, and believes that it is itself such a continuing entity" [33]. A newly born infant does not meet this requirement. Tooley does not endorse the gratuitous killing of children, but in weighing options (say, a seriously handicapped child who would make the parents' life extremely difficult), there may be extreme cases in which it is acceptable to kill the child.

Peter Singer argues to similar effect. In his words, "a week-old baby is not a rational and self-aware being, and there are many non human animals whose rationality, self-awareness, capacity to feel and so on, exceed that of a human baby a week or a month old. If... the fetus does not have the same claim to life as a person, it appears that the newborn baby does not either" [34]. Singer suggests that there are circumstances in which infanticide might be morally justified. For example, he argues that if a newborn infant is severely disabled and would have a very low quality of life, it may be more humane to end the infant's life than to subject them to a lifetime of suffering.

Presumably, both Tooley and Singer would agree that the trolley ought not to be diverted, since four fetuses do not outweigh the moral status of one adult person.

Tooley and Singer's position strikes many people as extreme. But it is also important to consider that the stringent anti-abortion view that would ultimately place more value on five embryos on a petri dish over one adult person, is also extreme. Some balancing point must surely exist, although it is by no means easy to find such a point. Considering the two trolley scenarios presented above (and presumably, most people's responses to such dilemmas), it does seem as if before ninety days, the fetus has no moral status, but at nine months of gestation, it is a much more difficult call. This may not suffice in terms of precision, but at least it is enough to uphold the morality of abortions in the early phases.

## Abortion as an Act of Self-defense

In discussing the ethics of self-defense and the bombing of abortion clinics, I have raised the idea of fetuses as victims—hence the appeal to stop an ongoing genocide. But it is also possible to think of fetuses as aggressors, and pregnant mothers as victims. It is important to consider the many ways in which a fetus represents a menace to the mother's well-being.

The process of being pregnant and giving birth comes with risks ranging from minor discomforts to severe complications that can be life threatening. Even though medical advancements have reduced maternal mortality rates in parts of the world, pregnancy and childbirth still present dangers to women's health. Gestational diabetes is a form of diabetes that develops during pregnancy and can lead to complications for both the pregnant woman and the fetus [35]. If left untreated or poorly managed, gestational diabetes can increase the risk of high blood pressure and predispose the mother to type 2 diabetes later in life. Hypertensive disorders of pregnancy, including gestational hypertension, preeclampsia, and eclampsia, involve high blood pressure and can have serious consequences for maternal and fetal health [36]. Preeclampsia is a leading cause of maternal and perinatal morbidity and mortality worldwide [37]. Eclampsia, a severe form of pre-eclampsia, can result in seizures, stroke, and other life-threatening complications if not promptly treated.

Pregnancy can also give rise to a variety of obstetric complications, including placental abnormalities [38]. umbilical cord problemsm, [39] and fetal malpresentations, which may necessitate medical interventions such as cesarean section or instrumental delivery (e.g., forceps or vacuum extraction). These complications can increase the risk of maternal and neonatal morbidity and may require close monitoring and specialized care during pregnancy and childbirth.

Even after delivery, women may suffer serious consequences as a result of pregnancy [40]. The postpartum period, extending from childbirth to the first few weeks or months after delivery, is associated with unique health challenges for the mother, including postpartum haemorrhage, [41] infections (e.g., uterine or wound infections), [42] breastfeeding difficulties, and mental health disorders such as postpartum depression and anxiety [43].

Some of these conditions would certainly be life-threatening. The causal agent is clearly the fetus. As per the tenets of self-defense ethics, is there moral authority to kill the fetus in self-defense?

Judith Jarvis Thomson considers the case of a villainous man driving a trolley towards you. What are you entitled to do? Thomson argues that even if you recognize the man as someone you deeply hate, you would still be entitled to take the necessary steps to avoid him from killing you. If that implies firing an antitank gun at the trolley, so be it. As she explains, "the driver is villainously aggressing against you, and will thereby kill you unless you stop him" [28].

A woman may hate the fetus she is carrying because, say, it was fathered by a man she deeply abhors. Pure hatred of the fetus may not be sufficient moral reason to kill it, but if the fetus seriously threatens her life, she is then entitled to act in self-defense. It just so happens that she hates the fetus, but that is not what provides moral justification. Rather, the defensive nature of her act does.

It is reasonable to posit that self-defense should be a last resort, employed only when no reasonable alternatives are available to avoid or mitigate the threat. In the trolley case, Thomson argues that if there is no need to blow up the trolley and you can stop it by other means, then that is what you ought to do. In her words, "it would be wrong to kill even a villainous aggressor when you do not need to do so" [28].

Likewise, self-defense is justified only when there is an imminent threat of harm. This means that the threat must be immediate and unavoidable, leaving no reasonable opportunity to escape or seek help. Acting in self-defense against a future or hypothetical threat, or when the threat has already passed, is unjustified. In the trolley scenario, the driver is heading towards you, so the threat is imminent.

Can the same be said about abortions? In many of the conditions specified above, the only effective way of preventing the harm done by the fetus is by killing it. Admittedly, prenatal care, medical treatment, monitoring and surveillance and even lifestyle changes can serve as palliatives in some conditions, but ultimately, the most serious threat can only be properly addressed with abortion. Likewise, the harm done by fetuses may not be as imminent as in the case of a villainous driver hurtling a trolley towards you, but in some circumstances, the harm done by the fetus may be so severe that, even while not immediately life-threatening, it does pose a significant risk.

It is important to accept two standards of imminence, depending on the context. In the case of a trolley hurtling towards you, imminence is indeed defined by the very short distance separating the trolley from your position. However, in the context of abortion (and medical procedures at large), the use of a wider concept of imminence is reasonable. As Eugene Volokh explains, "lethal self-defense is generally allowed only in response to imminent threats of harm, usually measured in minutes; medical self- defense would often be used to prevent deaths that are likely in months. But for medical self-defense, it makes sense to treat imminence as simply requiring a present life-threatening medical condition—that is to say, as a type of necessity requirement-not as requiring that death be likely within the hour" [44].

It is of course a matter of debate where the line must be drawn in terms of harm. Surely the ethics of self-defense are not only limited to life-threatening conditions. Some aggressions may be so severe that even while not threatening life itself, may warrant acts of self-defense from the victim. Suppose that the trolley driven by the villain is hurtling towards you, but it will only run over your legs, and you will likely survive. Does that invalidate your right to fire the antitank gun? Most people would say you are still entitled to fire the gun as an act of self-defense. Suppose now that the trolley driven by the evil man is hurtling towards the tracks located near you, and the only harm it will do is to splash the muddle on the tracks and stain your clothes. In that case, would you have the right to fire the antitank gun? Hardly.

As applied to abortion, it is difficult to stipulate which conditions resemble more the first or second trolley scenarios. Perhaps an analogue to general self-defense laws is in order. As Eileen McDonagh explains, "the latitude for the use of deadly force in self-defense in our culture and legal system extends beyond threats to one's life alone and includes threats of serious bodily injury and the loss of liberty, as in rape, kidnapping, or slavery" [45].

McDonagh further makes the case as follows: "Even in a medically normal pregnancy, the fetus massively intrudes on a woman's body and expropriates her liberty. If a woman does not consent to this transformation and use of her body, the fetus's imposition constitutes injuries sufficient to justify the use of deadly force to stop it." This line of argument may be extreme, but McDonagh does point her finger onto a reasonable point: the fetus' aggression goes beyond life-or-death situations.

Most legislation concurs that, in extreme situations where the mother's life is at risk, abortion is allowed [46]. However, the most stringent anti-abortion positions do not even allow for this. For example, direct abortion, which is the intentional killing of the unborn child as an end or means, is considered morally impermissible in Catholic teaching under any circumstances.

It is important to understand the methods for direct abortion, so as to distinguish them from other procedures that may result in abortion, albeit indirectly [47]. For example, there may be surgical methods, such as vacuum aspiration, dilation and curettage, and dilation and evacuation. There may also be the administration of drugs (such as mifepristone and misoprostol) to induce abortion. This is different from some treatments of ectopic pregnancies or extraction of the uterus as treatment of cancer; in these cases, the fetus may die, but the procedure does not target the fetus directly.

Catholic teaching does allow the use of indirect methods, on the basis of the principle of double effect (more of which, later), but it is quite strict in disapproving of direct abortions, even in cases where both the fetus and the mother's lives are at risk if the pregnancy is not terminated [48]. The grounding of this stance is that the fetus, even if it has the potential to cause harm, can never be considered an aggressor. From the perspective of Catholic moral theology, the fetus is not considered an aggressor but rather an innocent human being deserving of protection and care.

This stringent anti-abortion position seems to be founded upon the idea that on account of its own nature, the fetus is intrinsically innocent, and therefore, deserves no harm. Yet, this is a largely misguiding principle, as in the ethics of self-defense, the intent of the aggressor is ultimately irrelevant. Recall that the goal of the self-defense act is to impede the aggression, not to punish the aggressor. Ultimately, what matters is the act of aggression itself, not the intent (or even the character) of the aggressor.

Consider another trolley dilemma presented by Thomson. This time, the trolley is hurtling towards you, but "the driver is entirely without fall for what he is doing... some villain had injected him with a drug that made him go temporarily crazy... he is not villainously aggressing against you; but he is aggressing against you" [28]. Thomson calls the driver in this trolley scenario an "innocent aggressor."

As a result of pregnancy, a woman may suffer from diabetes, and this is a major risk to her life. Is the fetus at fault? No, the fetus is entirely innocent. But that does not protect it from actions pursued under the justification of self-defense. Thomson acknowledges that, in some cases, the extent of culpability of the aggressor may determine how the act of self-defense is pursued. For example, she writes: "Suppose an aggressor will take, not both your legs, but only your left foot unless you kill him. Here the aggressor's fault or lack of fault may well be thought to make a difference: thus it may be thought that you may kill him to defend your left foot against his aggression if he is at fault but not if he is without fault" [28]. This implies that when the aggression comes from an innocent being, the threshold for justification of self-defense is higher. In terms of abortion, given the innocence of the fetus, it would not be sufficient to justify killing the fetus simply because of some minor headache during pregnancy. But as explained above, pregnancy can have many more severe consequences (some of them life-threatening) and in those cases, the innocence of the fetus is irrelevant.

This trolley scenario also serves to understand the so-called "insanity defense" upheld by forensic psychiatrists and many legal scholars [49]. As per the M'Naughten rule, a person is legally insane and not responsible for their actions if, at the time of the crime, they were suffering from a mental illness or defect that rendered them unable to understand the nature and quality of their actions or unable to distinguish right from wrong [50]. This implies that the person is rendered not guilty of the crime. It is important to notice that the M'Naughten rule applies only once the aggressor has been detained and taken to court. It certainly does not apply while the person is in the middle of the aggression itself; while it may be that the person is not responsible for what she is doing, the potential victims of the aggression are entitled to act in self-defense. The culpability of the aggressor is immaterial in those circumstances.

Nevertheless, the trolley scenario presented by Thomson may not serve as an adequate analogy to abortion, because the fetus is not itself an agent taking steps to cause harm to the victim. Recall that in this trolley scenario, the driver is called "innocent aggressor." The driver is innocent to the extent that, very much as the person acquitted on the basis of the insanity defense, does not act out of her own demeanor or free will. Nevertheless, the innocent aggressor is at the origin of the aggression and has taken the necessary steps to begin the aggression.

That is not the case with the fetus. The fetus may be causally involved in the act of aggression, but it is doubtful that it is an aggressor itself. The mother may suffer threatening conditions as a result of the pregnancy, but the fetus is not deliberately seeking to cause them. If anything, the fetus is part of the aggression, but not the aggressor itself. As opposed to what is depicted in the previous trolley dilemma, the fetus is not an innocent aggressor, but rather, an "innocent threat."

Robert Nozick defines it as follows: "an innocent threat is someone who innocently is a causal agent in a process such that he would be an aggressor had he chosen to become such an agent. If someone picks up a third party and throws him at you down at the bottom of a deep well, the third party is innocent and a threat; had he chosen to launch himself at you in that trajectory he would be an aggressor" [51].

Thomson elaborates on this thought experiment as follows: "You are lying in the sun on your deck. Up in the cliff-top park above your house, a fat man is sitting on a bench, eating a picnic lunch. A villain now pushes the fat man off the cliff down toward you. If you do nothing, the fat man will fall on you, and be safe. But he is very fat, so if he falls on you, he will squash you flat and thereby kill you. What alternative do you have? Well, you only have time to shift the position of your awning; if you do this, the fat man will be deflected away from you. But deflecting him away from you will be deflecting him past the edge of the deck down onto the road below. Does morality permit you to shift the awning" [28]? Both the fetus and the falling fat man in this dilemma are innocent threats; they are causally engaged in aggression, but they are not aggressors themselves.

Thomson argues that, even in a case like this, there is justification for self-defense. However, it is important to understand what is required for moral justification in the action. It is not merely a matter of survival. Thomson considers the following trolley scenario: "a villain has started a trolley down a track toward you, and the only way you have of defending yourself is to shoot a bystander who stands on a footpath over the track: he is sufficiently heavy to crush the trolley's roof-top mechanism when he falls onto it, which will thereby stop the trolley" [28]. In this case, you are acting in self-defense. But you are targeting a person who is neither an aggressor nor a threat. Although killing that person would save your own life, the person who is targeted is not at all involved in the aggression.

This is similar to an ancient dilemma known as the "plank of Carneades" [52, 53]. In this scenario, two individuals are stranded at sea with only one plank or raft that can support the weight of one person. If both individuals cling to the plank, it will sink, and both will drown. If one person pushes the other off the plank, she will survive but the other will drown. The dilemma arises from the conflict between self-preservation and moral responsibility. The person pushed off from the plank is not causally participant in the drowning of the other person; therefore, she is not even an innocent threat. The scenario illustrates that self-preservation is different from self-defense. There is moral authority to act upon the principles of the latter, but not the former.

However, the fetus is causally participating in the aggression towards the mother. The falling fat man has no bad intentions and is only an unwilling passive participant in the aggression, but is a participant, nevertheless. That person is not at fault. But Thomson posits an irrelevance-of-fault-to-permissibility thesis: "it is irrelevant to the question whether X may do alpha whether X would be at fault doing it" [28]. This also applies to intention.

The falling fat man has a right not to be killed and is not at fault, and neither does he have full agency in the aggression. But in Thomson's reasoning, rights can sometimes be infringed without being violated, even if no fault has been committed. Thomson argues that whenever someone is part of the aggression, that person has violated another person's right, and their own right not to be killed can be infringed, since "agency is not required for violation of a right" [28]. The right not to be killed is absolute, only when it pertains to not being killed unjustly. But sometimes, you can be killed justly, even if you commit no fault. Being part of an aggression (regardless of intent or agency) makes you liable to lose the right not to be killed, and you would still be killed justly.

Now, as per Thomson's reasoning, once a person has lost the right not to be killed, she has no right to fight back. This is a bullet Thomson is prepared to bite. She explains: "I suggest that the permissibility of X's killing Y in self-defense goes hand in hand with the impermissibility of Y's fighting back" [28]. Of course, nobody expects a fetus to fight back in abortion. But the moral impermissibility of the fetus' prospect in fighting back serves to clarify Thomson's account of self-defense: you can be targeted once your right to not be killed has been forfeited (again, even if you are faultless and have no agency in the aggression).

The abortion debate is frequently framed in terms of rights. Those who uphold the pro-choice position typically focus on the moral status and personhood of the fetus. While acknowledging the biological humanity of the fetus, pro-choice advocates may argue that personhood is a complex and multifaceted concept that goes beyond biological existence. They may assert that personhood entails attributes such as consciousness, self-awareness, and the capacity for experiences, which may not be present in early stages of fetal development. In contrast, pro-life advocates insist that the fetus' moral status warrants it a right to life.

Thomson's account of self-defense makes this debate largely irrelevant. It may be granted that the fetus has a right to life, very much as any other adult. But as the above thought experiments show, this right is not absolute: in those cases, even an adult's right to life can be forfeited (either the villainous aggressor, the innocent aggressor, or the falling fat man). If the fetus is part of an aggression (regardless of its fault or agency), then its right to life can be forfeited in the attempt to stop that aggression.

Thomson's views have been challenged, most notably by Otsuka [54]. He posits that there is a moral equivalence between killing a bystander in the attempt to stop the trolley and killing the falling fat man. Recall that Thomson argues that the bystander has no involvement whatsoever in the aggression, whereas the falling fat man is an innocent threat for whom, even while faultless, the right not to be killed has been forfeited given his causal role in the aggression. Otsuka, in contrast, argues that there is no relevant difference between them.

In order to make his case, Otsuka presents the following scenario: "First imagine that an innocent person is lying alongside the path of a runaway trolley car. Unless you hurl at that trolley a bomb that you know will also kill the innocent person, the trolley will run you over" [54]. This is a case of an innocent bystander, and Otsuka concurs that in this case there is no justification in killing. Otsuka then presents a second scenario: "Now imagine a second case in which the same person is trapped inside a runaway trolley car. Unless you hurl a bomb that would destroy the trolley, and hence also the innocent person, the trolley will run you over before coming to a gentle stop" [54].

Otsuka makes the claim that "if doing that which foreseeably will kill the person is impermissible in the case in which the person is alongside the trolley, then I do not see how it could be permissible if the person is inside the trolley" [54]. Otsuka's rationale for this position is that "changing the location of the person should not make any moral difference" [54].

This is plausible, as indeed, in both cases, the person is not causally involved in the aggression, and their exact location would be irrelevant. But Otsuka then goes on to argue that in a case such as the one in which a person is tied to the front of the trolley and the impact of her body will kill you, you are not morally authorized to fire the gun. He further explains that "the only factual difference between the second case [the person riding inside the trolley] and the third [the falling fat man] that might lend support to the claim that it is permissible to kill in the third case but not the second is that in the third case it is the person's body that will kill you, whereas, in the second case, it is rather the trolley in which the person is encased that will kill you" [54]. Indeed, that has been Thomson's point all along. Although there is a difference in location, it is not the location itself what matters. What truly matters is the causal link: in the second case, the person is not part of the aggression; in the third case, he *is* part of the aggression. The extent to which the person participates in the aggression does matter. Admittedly, in both cases, there is a lack of control, as both persons have no control of the trolley. But again, control (or agency) is not what matters; what matters is participation in the causal chain of aggression, regardless of responsibility. The bystander is not bound to kill you, the person attached to the front of the trolley is.

Otsuka finds the following situation counterintuitive: "even if it would, for example, be impermissible to kill a falling person if it were only the mass of the enormous sky boots attached to her feet that would kill you, it would be permissible to kill her if it were, instead, the mass of her body that would kill you" [54]. Whether or not most people find this counterintuitive needs to be empirically assessed. But it does seem that most people have the intuition that one must follow the causal chain in justifying self-defense, and this ultimately implies that, indeed, if solely the boots are bound to kill you, then you may not kill the person; in contrast, if the person's body itself is included in the causal chain to kill you, then you may kill the person in self-defense.

Otsuka even goes to the extreme of asserting that innocent aggressors ought not to be killed in self-defense. Recall that trolley scenario: the trolley is going towards you, but its driver has been drugged by a villain to go temporarily crazy. Again, given that his justification focuses on control, then Otsuka naturally concludes that to the extent that the innocent aggressor has no control over what he is doing, his right to not be killed has not been forfeited.

This reasoning has implausible implications. Admittedly, a person who has no rational control of her own actions cannot be justifiably blamed for such actions, and indeed, that is the whole point of the insanity defense. But surely that is not a good argument not to stop someone from killing another person, in the midst of the aggression. Even in successful appeals to the insanity defense, the mentally unfit person must be kept within security bounds, precisely in order to avoid further harm to others. Otsuka claims that, on the basis of numbers (i.e., one aggressor threatening the life of many people), innocent aggressors must be stopped; they would only be protected from self-defense actions if there were only one victim. But this is still not a satisfactory caveat. A person has a right not to be killed; once that person is causally engaged in an act of aggression against someone else (again, regardless of the control over the action), that right is forfeited.

Thomson applied this reasoning explicitly to the issue of abortion, in perhaps her most famous piece of writing, "A Defense of Abortion." In discussing cases of self-defense, we have taken for granted that the scenario pertains to life-or-death or at least some considerable injury, and this would be analogous to high-risk pregnancies. But what about normal pregnancies? There is no significant threat to the mother's life. At most, normal pregnancies entail some measure of inconvenience for nine months.

Thomson argues that even in such cases, the fetus' moral status is irrelevant. While not an aggressor, the fetus is still a transgressor, in the sense that it invades the woman's own bodily space. The mother is not morally required to host it.

Thomson proposes a famous thought experiment in order to illustrate her point: "You wake up in the morning and find yourself back to back in bed with an unconscious violinist. A famous unconscious violinist. He has been found to have a fatal kidney ailment, and the Society of Music Lovers has canvassed all the available medical records and found that you alone have the right blood type to help. They have therefore kidnapped you, and last night the violinist's circulatory system was plugged into yours, so that your kidneys can be used to extract poisons from his blood as well as your own. The director of the hospital now tells you, "Look, we're sorry the Society of Music Lovers did this to you—we would never have permitted it if we had known. But still, they did it, and the violinist is now plugged into you. To unplug you would be to kill him. But never mind, it's only for nine months. By then he will have recovered from his ailment, and can safely be unplugged from you." Is it morally incumbent on you to accede to this situation" [55]?

Thomson argues that in a situation like this, there is no such moral requirement. The violinist has a right to live, but the obligation does not fall on you to save him. It would be heroic for you to volunteer, but you would not be unjust if you refused.

As applied to abortion, this reasoning implies that even if the fetus is a person, it is not the mother's duty to provide her body for purposes of gestation. Thomson emphasizes that she is not denying the fetus' right to a life; she is "arguing only that having a right to life does not guarantee having either a right to be given the use of or a right to be allowed continued use of another person's body—even if one needs it for life itself" [55].

Most legislation throughout the world seems to acknowledge at least part of this reasoning. After all, even in territories where abortion is criminalized, some exceptions for cases of rape are allowed [56]. There is some at least tacit understanding that rape is a heinous act of violence that violates a woman's bodily autonomy and right to consent, and therefore she is not morally required to carry on with the pregnancy. Unlike consensual sexual encounters where both parties willingly engage, rape involves coercion, force, or manipulation, and the woman does not voluntarily consent to the act that leads to pregnancy. Such legislation weighs the rights of the woman, who is a victim of a violent crime, against the rights of the unborn child, recognizing that the circumstances of conception were involuntary and traumatic.

Yet, Thomson argues that in terms of moral requirement to carry on the pregnancy, there is no relevant difference between being raped and not being raped. In her words, "surely the question of whether you have a right to life at all, or how much of it you have, shouldn't turn on the question of whether or not you are a product of a rape" [55]. It might be argued that whether or not rape took place is relevant, because once a woman consents to a sexual act, she must take responsibility for the consequences of that act. By consenting to sex, she has—so to speak— opened the gates of her body to an outsider, and now it is her duty to serve as a host.

But Thomson offers an effective reply. She argues: "if the room is stuffy, and I therefore open a window to air it, and a burglar climbs in, it would be absurd to say, "Ah, now he can stay, she's given him a right to the use of her house—for she is partially responsible for his presence there, having voluntarily done what enabled him to get in, in full knowledge that there are such things as burglars, and that burglars burgle"" [55].

Furthermore, it may very well be the case that women take precautions to avoid pregnancy, but such measures still fail. For example, a woman may forget to take birth control pills at the same time every day, or it may be that condoms are not used correctly (e.g., incorrect placement, failure to use throughout the entire sexual encounter), or not following instructions for other contraceptive methods accurately. Additionally, each contraceptive method has a failure rate, which represents the percentage of women who will become pregnant within the first year of using the method, even with correct and consistent use [57]. No contraceptive method is 100% effective. Likewise, certain medications, supplements, or substances (e.g., antibiotics, anticonvulsants) can interfere with the effectiveness of hormonal contraceptives like birth control pills, patches, or rings, reducing their efficacy [58]. Even some health conditions or medical procedures, such as vomiting or diarrhea (which can affect the absorption of oral contraceptives), bariatric surgery (which can affect the absorption of medications), or certain gastrointestinal disorders, may impact the effectiveness of contraceptive methods.

This discussion goes back to a point discussed in the previous chapter: supererogatory actions. These are actions that go beyond what is morally required or expected of an individual. These actions are considered praiseworthy, virtuous, or admirable but are not obligatory. In other words, they are acts that are above and beyond the call of duty. They are typically acts that entail sacrificing one's own interests or well-being to help others in need, even when there is no obligation to do so.

It would be nice for you to stay plugged in to the violinist for nine months, but such an action would only be supererogatory, not morally required. Likewise, even if her life is not in danger, a woman's willingness to lend her body for nine months for the gestation of a fetus is an act of supererogation.

Most legislation tacitly acknowledges that there are acts that, while it would be good for citizens to do, are not required to be done, and therefore, there is no penalty for such omissions. There are very few so-called "Bad Samaritan" laws, and where they exist, they remain very controversial [59–61]. These are statutes that impose a legal obligation on individuals to provide assistance to others in distress or in need of help, typically in emergency situations. These laws aim to encourage bystanders to intervene and provide aid when someone's life or well-being is at risk. As it is well-known, the term "Bad Samaritan" is derived from the biblical parable in which a Samaritan helps a traveler who has been beaten and left for dead on the side of the road, while others pass by without offering assistance.

Many legal scholars have long argued against these statues. On the same principle as Thomson's argument, many critics raise concerns about the infringement of individual rights and freedoms inherent in Bad Samaritan laws. Mandating individuals to do acts of kindness may be seen as an undue intrusion into personal autonomy and freedom of choice. Critics argue that individuals should have the right to decide whether to engage in such acts based on their own assessment of risks, capabilities, and moral obligations, rather than being compelled to act by legal mandates.

Nevertheless, there may be extreme situations that do warrant some moral requirement to act. Some life-saving actions may come at such a small price, that refusing to do them may indeed be a major moral failure, perhaps with legal implications. For example, in one disturbing story, it is reported that a man in Florida "drowned in a pond while teens recorded and mocked him"; [62] for these teens, it would have taken very little effort to save the man's life yet refused to do it. Cases like this have prompted some legislators to reconsider passing Bad Samaritan laws.

Thomson herself acknowledges that her argument can only be considered as a matter of degree. If you only had to stay plugged in to the violinist for fifteen minutes in order to save his life, would there be a moral duty to do so in that case? As applied to the ethics of abortion, Thomson writes: "suppose pregnancy lasted only an hour, and constituted no threat to life or health. And suppose that a woman becomes pregnant as a result of rape. Admittedly she did not voluntarily do anything to bring about the existence of a child. Admittedly she did nothing at all which would give the unborn person a right to the use of her body. All the same it might well be said… that she ought to allow it to remain for that hour—that it would be indecent of her to refuse" [55].

Now, Thomson calls the situation "indecent", but she still refuses to call it "unjust." In her words, "even supposing a case in which a woman pregnant due to rape ought to allow the unborn person to use her body for the hour he needs, we should not conclude that he has a right to do so; we should say that she is self-centered, callous, indecent, but not unjust, if she refuses. The complaints are no less grave; they are just different" [55]. This would not just be a semantic issue. Someone who refuses to do a simple act of kindness with so many implications may deserve the scorn of people, but that is different from saying that such a person is morally required to do so.

Thomson favors the concept of a Minimally Decent Samaritan: by and large, people have the prerogative to choose not to act, but in some extreme circumstances, it would only be decent for them to do so. Thomson even thinks it would be a good idea to have laws enforcing this concept. She also applies this reasoning (but only in the moral realm, not the legal realm) to abortion: "while I do argue that abortion is not impermissible, I do not argue that it is always permissible. There may well be cases in which carrying the child to term requires only Minimally Decent Samaritanism of the mother, and this is a standard we must not fall below. I am inclined to think it a merit of my account precisely that it does not give a general yes or a general no. It allows for and supports our sense that, for example, a sick and desperately frightened fourteen-year-old schoolgirl, pregnant due to rape, may of course choose abortion, and that any law which rules this out is an insane law. And it also allows for and supports our sense that in other cases resort to abortion is even positively indecent. It would be indecent in the woman to request an abortion, and indecent in a doctor to perform it, if she is in her seventh month, and wants the abortion just to avoid the nuisance of postponing a trip abroad" [55].

However, the fact of the matter is that abortion still requires nine months, and for some women (especially those whose pregnancy is the result of rape), carrying the fetus inside their body until delivery may be too demanding. But things may change in the future due to technological advances. While it is unlikely that—as in Thomson's hypothetical scenario—pregnancies would only last one hour, the prospect of ectogenesis—artificial wombs—may be taken more seriously [63].

Of course, there are some important challenges. While there have been advancements in the development of artificial womb technology, particularly for supporting the growth and development of premature infants, the successful gestation of an embryo from the earliest stages of development (such as a 1-week embryo) to full term outside of a human body remains a distant prospect [64]. There are scientific challenges with replicating the first weeks of pregnancy accurately in an artificial setting. Mimicking the maternal–fetal interactions (in terms of providing essential nutrients, oxygen, and immune support to the developing embryo) outside of the maternal body would require very advanced and sophisticated bioengineering techniques.

But the history of technology suggests that in many instances, what was once considered highly improbable may come to fruition in the future. If artificial wombs do become a reality and the embryo can be gestated artificially, say, within days of conception, then this may have relevant implications on the morality of abortion.

Some pro-life groups favor the slogan "Adoption is an option," [65] implying that instead of undergoing an abortion, women should carry the fetus to delivery, and then give it up for adoption. This is not sensible enough, as asking a victim of rape (or any other woman enduring difficulties during pregnancy) to carry on for nine months is too much. But in the future, it may well be reasonable to proclaim "ectogenesis is an option." If pregnancy could be shortened to, say, 24 h, then it may be an act of Minimally Decent Samaritanism for most women to wait until the embryo is extracted. Ectogenesis technology could weaken arguments based on bodily autonomy in favor of abortion. If a pregnant woman could opt for ectogenesis to transfer the embryo to an artificial womb, she might be seen as having a way to avoid the bodily burdens of pregnancy while still allowing the fetus to develop.

Ultimately, the point in defending abortion is to liberate women from the burden of a foreign agent invading the body, not to gratuitously kill the fetus. Even people on the pro-choice side of this debate would agree with this concession from Thomson: "while I am arguing for the permissibility of abortion in some cases, I am not arguing for the right to secure the death of the unborn child. It is easy to confuse these two things in that up to a certain point in the life of the fetus it is not able to survive outside the mother's body; hence removing it from her body guarantees its death. But they are importantly different… A woman may be utterly devastated by the thought of a child, a bit of herself, put out for adoption and never seen or heard of again. She may therefore want not merely that the child be detached from her, but more, that it die… I agree that the desire for the child's death is not one which anybody may gratify, should it turn out to be possible to detach the child alive" [55].

## The Doctrine of Double Effect

Even the most stringent opponents of abortion would agree that there are some morally acceptable medical procedures which may end in the death of the fetus. For example, in an ectopic pregnancy, the fertilized egg implants outside the uterus, usually in the fallopian tube [66]. This condition is life-threatening for the pregnant person as the pregnancy cannot develop normally and may lead to serious complications, including rupture of the fallopian tube and internal bleeding, which can be fatal. One common medical procedure in such cases is to remove the fallopian tubes of the pregnant woman, thus resulting in the death of the embryo.

Even people who claim that there is no moral justification to kill an innocent threat in self-defense, would concede that, in this case, the procedure is within the bounds of morality. In order to see why, this case can be contrasted with craniotomy, the crushing of the fetus' brain in order to kill it. It seems one important moral difference between both cases is how direct the procedure is [67]. In craniotomy, the fetus is specifically targeted, and therefore, the intention is to kill the fetus. In contrast, in removing the fallopian tubes, the intention is merely to save the mother's life. If the fetus survives, the purpose is spoiled in craniotomy. If the embryo survives, the purpose is not spoiled in removing the fallopian tubes.

A similar reasoning can be applied to cases of euthanasia. Consider two cases of actions that result in a patient's death. First, a physician decides to alleviate a patient's severe pain by injecting a large dose of morphine. Ultimately, the effects of the morphine result in the patient's death. Second, a physician contemplates a patient's suffering, and decides that the best way to end it is by killing the patient. In order to do so, he injects a large dose of morphine.

Daniel Sumasy has a very useful question, as consideration of whether a particular action in end-of-life care is morally acceptable: "if the patient were not to die after my actions, would I feel that I had failed to accomplish what I had set out to do" [68]? In the first case, the answer to Sumasy's question is "no". If the patient survived the morphine injection, the physician would not have failed in his or her endeavor. The intention was not to kill the patient, but rather, to alleviate the pain. Death was not used as a means to bring about the alleviation of pain. Yes, the physician may foresee that the patient may die, but it was never intended. Even though the physician's actions amounted to killing the patient (not merely letting him or her die), this is not euthanasia per se, and it is morally acceptable as per the doctrine of double effect.

In contrast, in the second case, the answer to Sumasy's question is "yes". If the patient survived the morphine injection, the physician would have failed in the original endeavor. The intention was to kill the patient, as death was conceived of as a means to an end. The patient's death was not merely foreseen, it was intended.

This difference between intending and foreseeing is the foundation of the doctrine of double effect. Recall that, as per this doctrine, some actions that cause harm are allowed, but some requirements must be met. The action itself must be morally good or indifferent; the harm caused by the bad effect must not be disproportionate to the good achieved by the action, and there must be no other way to achieve the good effect without also causing the bad effect.

Additionally, the bad consequences of the act must be foreseen but not intended. When an individual intends a particular consequence, it means that she desires or aims for that consequence to occur as a result of their action. On the other hand, foreseeing a consequence means recognizing that a certain outcome is likely to occur as a result of one's actions, but not necessarily desiring or intending that outcome. If the bad consequence is directly intended, the action is morally impermissible; if the bad consequence is merely foreseen but not intended, the action may be morally permissible.

Although the doctrine of double effect has a long history in philosophy, [69] trolley scenarios have made it especially relevant. Thomson herself came up with a scenario which seems to provide a strong grounding to uphold the doctrine of double effect: "George is on a footbridge over the trolley tracks. He knows trolleys, and can see that the one approaching the bridge is out of control. On the track back of the bridge there are five people; the banks are so steep that they will not be able to get off the track in time. George knows that the only way to stop an out-of-control trolley is to drop a very heavy weight into its path. But the only available, sufficiently heavy weight is a fat man, also watching the trolley from the footbridge. George can shove the fat man onto the track in the path of the trolley, killing the fat man; or he can refrain from doing this, letting the five die" [70].

Thomson contrasted this dilemma with the scenario in which—as discussed in the previous chapter—a trolley is hurtling down a track towards five people who are tied up and unable to move, and a person is standing at a switch that can divert the trolley onto a different track where there is only one person tied up. Both cases imply killing one in order to save five. But the fundamental moral difference relates to the doctrine of double effect. George is using the fat man as a means to save the five; this implies that if somehow the fat man bounces off the track upon falling, his body would not stop the trolley, and that would defeat the purpose of the action. In contrast, in the scenario where the trolley is diverted, the death of the one person is not used as a means to save the five; should the man on the track manage to free himself and evade danger after altering the course of the trolley, the purpose would still be served. This outcome not only prevents a collision with the five individuals but also ensures no additional harm to anyone else.

Research in moral psychology has firmly documented that most people agree that there is a significant moral difference between both trolley dilemmas. In many surveys, whereas about 90% of subjects are willing to divert the trolley thus killing one and saving five, only about 12% of respondents are willing to push the fat man from the footbridge [71].

Yet, Thomson herself presented a variant of the dilemma that challenges the adequacy of the doctrine of double effect. In this version, a trolley is on its way to run five people; this time, it can be diverted on a separate track, but the diversion loops back to the main track, so that diverting the trolley will kill the five people. However, on the looping track there is a fat man tied to the track; when he is impacted by the trolley, his body will stop the trolley, and the five people will be saved [72]. Should the trolley be diverted?

This dilemma is seemingly very similar to the scenario in which the trolley must be diverted to save five and therefore killing one. Yet, in terms of the doctrine of double effect, there is a substantial difference. In the dilemma with the loop, the body of the fat man serves as a means to save the five. In the original trolley dilemma, if the one person tied to the track manages to escape, that would not defeat the purpose; in contrast, in the dilemma with the loop, if the fat man manages to escape, that would indeed defeat the purpose, as the other five persons would be killed. In this case, very much as in the scenario of the footbridge, the death of the fat man is not merely foreseen, but actually intended. As per the doctrine of double effect, the trolley should not be diverted, because that would entail using the fat man as a means and intending his death.

But Thomson insists that in this case, the trolley should be diverted to save the five, especially considering its similarity to the original trolley scenario. As she explains, "we cannot really suppose that the presence or absence of that extra bit of track makes a major difference as to what an agent may do in these cases, and it really does seem right to think (despite the discomfort) that the agent may proceed" [72].

Nevertheless, other experiments with trolley dilemmas suggest that, even in the case of the loop, the doctrine of double effect plays a role in moral decision-making. Consider this scenario presented by Marc Hauser: "Oscar is taking his daily walk near the trolley tracks when he notices that the trolley that is approaching is out of control. Oscar sees what has happened: The driver of the trolley saw five men walking across the tracks and slammed on the brakes, but the brakes failed and the driver fainted. The trolley is now rushing toward the five men. It is moving so fast that they will not be able to get off the track in time. Fortunately, Oscar is standing next to a switch, which he can throw, that will temporarily turn the trolley onto a side track. There is a heavy object on the side track. If the trolley hits the object, the object will slow the trolley down, thereby giving the men time to escape. Unfortunately, there is a man standing on the side track in front of the heavy object, with his back turned. Oscar can throw the switch, preventing the trolley from killing the men, but killing the man. Or he can refrain from doing this, letting the five die. Is it morally permissible for Oscar to throw the switch" [73]?

This case is similar to the scenario with the loop, but this time, the man is not used as a means to save the five. Hauser has found that the number of people who choose to kill the man in the dilemma with the loop is significantly (in statistical terms) lower than the number of people who choose to kill the man in Oscar's dilemma. On the basis of these results, Hauser concludes that "some forms of moral judgment are universal and mediated by unconscious and inaccessible principles", [71] and the doctrine of double effect may be one such principle.

However, other trolley dilemmas suggest that the doctrine of double effect is not altogether relevant in moral reasoning. Indeed, research in moral psychology indicates that in some of those dilemmas, people embrace the option that violates the doctrine of double effect. Consider, for example, a variant formulated by Joshua Greene and his collaborators. This case is similar to the trolley dilemma in which the fat man is thrown from the bridge, except that now, one "may drop the victim [the fat man] onto the tracks using a trap door" and a switch, and the switch is next to the fat man [74]. Greene's empirical study indicates that 59% of people favor pushing the switch in this situation. This is considerably higher than the responses in the original dilemma where the fat man is pushed from the bridge. An even higher percentage (63%) is obtained in a variant in which there is the option of dropping the fat man onto the tracks using a trap door, but this time, the switch is far from the action.

In both scenarios, the fat man is employed as a tool to rescue the five, with his collision with the trolley being deliberate. A strict adherence to the principle of double effect would need participants to eschew this choice. However, in these instances, most individuals are willing to sacrifice the fat man. This suggests that moral instincts concerning the principle of double effect are somewhat erratic, rendering it an unreliable moral compass.

It appears that whatever intuitive judgments are made regarding the doctrine of double effect, they are complicated by another factor that also influences outcomes: the use of direct physical force. Employing the overweight individual as a means to rescue five people elicits moral aversion (as seen in the footbridge scenario), yet the absence of direct physical force mitigates that aversion in the remote switch scenarios, where there is notably higher acceptance when the doctrine of double effect is disregarded but direct physical force is absent.

However, whether or not direct physical force is utilized in causing harm is scarcely morally pertinent. Is a perpetrator of war crimes less culpable because they send prisoners to the gas chamber instead of personally executing them? As our technological society progresses, the necessity for direct physical force diminishes in many tasks. Nonetheless, this does not absolve us of moral responsibility for our actions. Whether euthanasia, abortion, or any other controversial medical procedures are deemed morally acceptable should not hinge on whether the physician does the procedure with their own hands, administers a medication, or triggers a mechanism from a remote location.

Moreover, studies have shown that various factors complicate individuals' moral deliberations in trolley problem scenarios, many of which are unrelated to the doctrine of double effect. One such factor is framing effects. Empirical evidence indicates that the language used to present trolley dilemmas can impact participants' responses. For instance, in a study where the emphasis was placed on saving the five individuals rather than on the death of the one, participants were more inclined to endorse the utilitarian choice [75]. The order in which dilemmas are presented also has an effect on responses [76].

The morality of many medical procedures is frequently judged on the basis of the doctrine of double effect, and in turn, this doctrine is allegedly sustained by our moral intuitions. But the cases discussed above suggest that such intuitions are not (at least entirely) about the distinction between unintended and foreseen effects, or about the means/end relationship. Therefore, the support of the doctrine of double effect is not as robust as it may at first seem.

If the intuitions of most people are correct, then these results suggest that the doctrine of double effect is not altogether relevant in making these types of moral decisions. For, that would entail that, very much as most people are reluctant to push the fat man from the bridge, most people would be reluctant to divert the trolley with the loop; yet that is not the case (even if, as Hauser's study shows, the number of people willing to divert the trolley in the case of the loop is lower than in the case of Oscar).

Some philosophers have tried to salvage the doctrine of double effect and have countered that, despite intuitions, in the case of the loop it is wrong to divert the trolley. For example, Jeff McMahan writes as follows: "This intuition about the loop case has always been alien to me. Diverting the trolley in this case seems to me virtually indistinguishable morally from using the man to stop the trolley [in the dilemma of throwing the fat man from the footbridge]" [77]. He insists that it is not acceptable to turn the trolley in the dilemma with the loop. To make his case, he presents a variant of the dilemma with the loop as follows: "Suppose that after throwing the switch to divert the trolley, the bystander in the loop case discovers that it is possible to free the person on the branch track before he will be hit by the trolley… Ought she to free him? If she had this option in the original case, she would clearly be required to free him. But in the loop-option case she needs his body to stop the trolley. Suppose she refuses to free him. How is this relevantly different from placing the man in the path of the trolley [as in the dilemma with the footbridge]…? In both cases the bystander kills a man as a means of stopping the trolley" [77]. McMahan insists that his intuition is that "if she directs a trolley toward an innocent person, she must enable him to get out of its path, if she can, even if she thereby loses the opportunity to save the five" [77].

Perhaps philosophers such as McMahan would fear that if one morally endorses diverting the trolley in the scenario with the loop, then there would be no good reason to morally object to pushing the fat man from the footbridge. But whereas the doctrine of double effect would disapprove of killing one to save the five in both scenarios, Thomson believes that there is an important moral principle that serves to differentiate them. For Thomson, the morality of actions is guided by respect for rights.

Thomson argues that although in the scenario with the loop the fat man is used as a means, the fat man's rights are not violated, since diverting the trolley is not creating a new threat to him, but rather, merely redirecting an existing threat. This is different from the scenario of the footbridge, since there, by pushing the fat man a new threat is created, not merely redirected. Consequently, in the trolley dilemma with the loop, the fat man's rights are not violated, since he is already there, and all we are doing is redirecting an already existing threat; in contrast, in the dilemma with the footbridge, the fat man's rights are indeed violated, since we are initiating a new action.

Empirical research in moral psychology suggests that most people's intuitions fit along those lines. For example, one important study concludes that "moral intuitions are influenced by the locus of the intervention in the underlying causal model. In moral dilemmas, judgments conforming to the prescriptions of utilitarianism are more likely when the intervention influences the path of the agent of harm (e.g., the trolley) than when the intervention influences the path of the potential patient (i.e., victim)", or as the authors poetically express it, there is a difference between throwing a bomb on a person and throwing a person on a bomb [78].

However, Thomson's appeal to rights has problems of its own, to the extent that some other trolley dilemmas suggest that the relevant moral principle is not strictly upholding a person's rights. For example, Frances Kamm presents this trolley scenario: "Suppose that a trolley is headed toward five people who are seated on a large swivel table. Although we physically cannot redirect the trolley, we can swivel the table and save the five people. However, we thereby start a rock slide that will kill one innocent bystander… Here we start a new threat, rather than redistribute an existing one, and it kills someone" [79]. To the extent that a new threat was introduced, and it killed the innocent bystander, this would be a violation of his rights.

But Kamm insists that "it is permissible to swivel the table, and for the same reason that it is permissible to redirect the trolley" [79].

The reason Kamm appeals to is what she calls the "principle of permissible harm," and she defines it as follows: "It is permissible to cause harm to some in the course of achieving the greater good of saving a greater number of others from comparable harm, if the events which produce the greater good are not more intimately causally related to the production of harm than they are to the production of the greater good" [80].

In following this principle, she attempts to modify the doctrine of double effect, so that it can still be properly used in trolley scenarios such as the one with the loop. In her version of the doctrine, however, apart from the two effects that are frequently distinguished (intended vs. foreseen), Kamm posits that "there is a general conceptual distinction between doing something because it will have an effect and doing it in order to produce an effect" [79]. This moral rule is now known as the "doctrine of triple effect," and rests on the premise that the reasons for which someone acts are not necessarily the same as that person's intentions. This would allow the possibility that someone might take an action because it leads to a particular unfortunate event, even without the intention for that final outcome.

This may be a nice way to safeguard the doctrine of double effect, but in medicine, it does seem as if, sometimes, it may be morally acceptable to do some direct harm in order to achieve some greater purpose. Consider conjoined twins. In many cases, the separation of conjoined twins comes at the expense of killing one of them. As we have seen, the application of the doctrine of double effect states that the most relevant distinction is whether the bad effect is intended or merely foreseen. In the case of attempts at separating conjoined twins, it is not clear what the nature of the harmful effect is.

For example, in the notorious case of Mary and Jodie—conjoined twins born in 2000 in Malta—, they were joined at the pelvis, sharing a spinal column and lower digestive system. They had separate hearts, but Jodie's heart provided circulation for both twins. The twins were taken to England for treatment. Doctors anticipated that if they were not separated, both twins would die in a span of about six months. The medical team recommended the surgery and anticipated that in the procedure Mary would die. The twins' parents were devoutly Catholic and did not approve— they sought council from clergy and were advised not to carry on the procedure. However, the courts ruled that the procedure had to be carried out, even against the parents' wishes. The surgery was done, and as expected, Mary died, and Jodie survived.

Many Catholic commentators have indicated that the doctrine of double effect did not necessarily preclude the surgery. For example, Daniel Sulmasy explained: "in a real sense, examining the case from Mary's point of view, Jodie is Mary's life-support, not just her ventilator, but her heart and circulation as well. The church teaches that Mary, and those who speak for her, have no moral obligation to continue heroic measures to keep Mary alive. The effort to do so imposes profound burdens on Mary, and profound burdens on Jodie as well... Catholic moralists would not demand that Jodie sacrifice herself in order to keep her sister alive for a few more months" [81].

But as per another interpretation—the one favored by the clergy who counseled the parents—, this surgery did indeed violate the doctrine of double effect, because in separating the twins and detaching the weak twin (Mary) from the strong twin (Jodie), one is effectively seeking the former's death, and therefore, it is an intended result, and not merely foreseen.

For the sake of argument, let us suppose that the second interpretation is the correct one: the surgery is incompatible with the doctrine of double effect. Does that imply the surgery must not be carried out? This matter is open to debate, but considering that otherwise both twins would die, would it not better to save at least one of them? Is there a point in following the doctrine of double effect if everybody dies in the end? In the footbridge scenario, if the fat man is not pushed, he would not die. But imagine a scenario in which the fat man would die regardless. In that case, would it not be better to push the fat man so that at least we can save the five persons tied to the tracks? It is an open question.

In a famous debate, Bernard Williams charged against utilitarianism by claiming that this doctrine entails alienating a man "in a real sense from his actions and the source of his action in his own convictions. It is to make him into a channel between the input of everyone's projects, including his own, and an output of optimific decision; but this is to neglect the extent to which his projects and his decisions have to be seen as the actions and decisions which flow from the projects and attitudes with which he is most closely identified. It is thus, in the most literal sense, an attack on his integrity" [82].

Williams illustrated his argument through the story of Jim, a man faced with a harrowing moral dilemma in South America. Jim is presented with a stark choice: he can personally kill one native, or if he refuses, a soldier will execute twenty natives, including the one Jim could save by taking the single life. This conundrum is not unlike that of the conjoined twins. If they all will die regardless, would it not be better if at least some lives were saved? Williams encourages us to understand the profound difficulty of Jim's predicament, regardless of the choice he ultimately makes. He emphasizes that sacrificing one's personal integrity, even for ostensibly noble causes like saving lives, can erode the genuineness of one's moral principles. So, both for Jim and the twins' parents, whatever decision is made turns out to be very difficult, and if indeed they carry forward the plan to kill one to save others, that would affect their integrity. Nevertheless, Williams does not provide a definitive answer to the dilemma posed by Jim and the natives but uses it to highlight the complexities of moral decision-making and the importance of maintaining integrity even in difficult situations. Perhaps in some extreme situations the doctrine of double effect ought to be waived, but we must be prepared to acknowledge that those situations are profoundly regretful, and we should never feel too comfortable in deciding one way or the other.

# The Intricacies of Personhood and Abortion

In presenting trolley scenarios to discuss the ethics of abortion, I have made similes between the fetus (or embryo), and a person tied to the track, a fat man thrown from a bridge, and so on. Consequently, in these discussions about the ethics of killing, I have tacitly acknowledged that the fetus may very well be a person. One of Thomson's most forceful points is that whether the fetus is actually a person is largely irrelevant in making the case for the morality of abortion.

Nevertheless, this is an issue that still needs to be considered. At the beginning of this chapter, in discussing the morality of bombing abortion clinics, I have indirectly concluded that, at least in the initial phases of gestation, the fetus is not a person. However, a more direct examination is in order.

Those who oppose abortion assert that from the moment of conception, the fetus possesses a unique genetic identity distinct from its parents, marking the beginning of a new human life [83]. It is often argued that this genetic identity distinguishes the developing embryo or fetus as an individual human being with its own inherent worth and dignity. By highlighting the presence of human DNA in the zygote (the fertilized egg), pro-life proponents argue that from the earliest stages of development, the embryo possesses the genetic blueprint that defines it as a member of the human species [84]. They contend that this genetic makeup establishes the moral significance of the embryo or fetus.

Furthermore, in their understanding, embryology highlights the continuous development and growth of the fetus from the earliest stages of conception to birth; this developmental continuum underscores the continuity of the organism's life and its inherent value at every stage of development [85]. Likewise, people on the pro-life side of the debate emphasize the unity of the developing organism, wherein all the components necessary for the organism's development and growth are present from the earliest stages; in their view, this unity establishes the fetus as a distinct and whole human being deserving of moral consideration [86]. They also point out that there is a biological continuity between different stages of human development, from conception to adulthood; this sustains the moral consistency in protecting human life at all stages of development [87].

However, an important reply is that while the fetus may possess a unique genetic identity, personhood and moral status are not solely determined by genetic composition. Factors such as consciousness, self-awareness, and the ability to experience pain and pleasure are more relevant in determining moral status. Throughout most of gestation, the fetus lacks the neurological development necessary to experience sensations or emotions. Without consciousness, the fetus cannot possess preferences, desires, or interests that would warrant moral consideration.

Opponents of abortion frequently frame this conversation by referring to embryos as "innocent children." But is the embryo more similar to an egg or sperm, or to a baby? In determining moral status, it is important to consider sentience and consciousness. Since embryos lack these cognitive capacities, they may be considered akin to biological material rather than fully realized individuals with rights and interests comparable to those of a child. Embryos represent an early stage of the developmental process, and their moral significance increases as they develop more advanced neurological and cognitive functions; but it is important to realize that, at least in the early phases, the traits that endow a being with personhood are fundamentally lacking.

It is implausible to claim that the fetus retains some form of consciousness in the early phases of gestation, given what we know about the progression of pregnancies. Brain waves become detectable only by the eighth week, [88] but it is important to note that their mere presence is not sufficient to assure conscious experience. For sensations of pain (a fundamental aspect in any consideration of moral status) there must also be neural pathways that convey pain signals to the cerebral cortex. These neural pathways typically do not reach sufficient development until twenty to twenty-four weeks into gestation, [89] rendering pain perception highly improbable much before the conclusion of the second trimester.

In this context, it is important to distinguish between being a human and being a person. In the biological sense, "human being" simply refers to membership in the species *Homo sapiens*. From a biological perspective, a human fetus indisputably qualifies as a human being because it possesses human DNA and belongs to the species *Homo sapiens*. This sense of "human being" is purely descriptive and based on scientific classification. However, it is a mistake to assume that this biological classification is equated with moral personhood or moral status. Moral personhood involves attributes such as consciousness, self-awareness, and the capacity for moral agency. While a fetus may be biologically human, it does not necessarily follow that it possesses the same moral status as a fully developed human being.

Mary Anne Warren asks: "Can it be established that genetic humanity is sufficient for moral humanity?", to which she responds: "I think that there are very good reasons for not defining the moral community in that way. I would like to suggest an alternative way of defining the moral community... The suggestion is simply that the moral community consists of all and only people, rather than all and only human beings" [90]. Admittedly, the fetus is a human being, but it does not yet belong to the moral community of people, on account of its lack of attributes that define personhood.

Under the pro-choice view, personhood emerges when an individual becomes capable of subjective experiences, self-reflection, and awareness of their own existence. Personhood is also associated with the capacity for rational thought, moral decision-making, and the ability to engage in complex social relationships. These cognitive and moral capacities distinguish persons from other living beings and confer moral status and rights; individuals capable of reasoning, making choices, and understanding moral principles are typically considered persons deserving of respect and protection. Furthermore, the ability to experience sensations, emotions, and pleasure or pain is also significant; entities capable of subjective experiences, such as feeling pleasure or suffering, may be accorded greater moral consideration than those lacking such capacities.

And very much as embryos are human beings but not persons, there may be persons who are not human beings. For example, extraterrestrial life forms may have different evolutionary histories, physiologies, or modes of consciousness that challenge conventional definitions of personhood based on human attributes. Warren considers the case as follows: "Imagine a space traveler who lands on an unknown planet and encounters a race of beings utterly unlike any he has ever seen or heard of. If he wants to be sure of behaving morally toward these beings, he has to somehow decide whether they are people, and hence have full moral rights, or whether they are the sort of thing which he need not feel guilty about treating as, for example, a source of food" [90]. Clearly, the moral status of those beings cannot be solely determined by whether or not they have, say, twenty-three pairs of chromosomes.

In light of the hard scientific evidence that indicates that fetuses do not have the neural capacity for consciousness, people on the pro-life side of the debate point to the fetus' potentiality [91]. This argument posits that the fetus possesses the inherent potential to develop into a fully formed human being, and therefore, it should be accorded the same moral status and rights as any other human being. As per this view, from the moment of conception, the fetus contains the genetic blueprint and developmental potential to grow and develop into a complete human being. To the extent that the fetus possesses the potential to become a fully realized human being, it should be granted the same moral consideration and rights as any other human being. Denying the fetus these rights would be equivalent to denying its inherent potential and devaluing its future existence.

In one of the most relevant indictments of the moral permissibility of abortion, Don Marquis expresses the argument as follows: "Premature death is a misfortune. Premature death is a misfortune, in general, because it deprives an individual of a future of value. An individual's future will be valuable to that individual if that individual will come, or would come, to value it. We know that killing us is wrong. What makes killing us wrong, in general, is that it deprives us of a future of value. Thus, killing someone is wrong, in general, when it deprives her of a future like ours" [92].

But it is important to note that potential rights differ from actual rights in that they are contingent upon the fulfillment of certain conditions. Certainly, a medical student is a potential doctor, but in no way does that imply that the student ought to be given the right to perform surgery on patients. The student still has a long way to go.

Michael Tooley illustrates this point with a thought experiment: "Suppose at some future time a chemical were to be discovered which when injected into the brain of a kitten would cause the kitten to develop into a cat possessing a brain of the sort possessed by humans, and consequently into a cat having all the psychological capabilities characteristic of adult humans. Such cats would be able to think, to use language, and so on" [33]. In that case, the transformed cats would be persons. But if the newborn kitten is killed, that is not as morally transgressive as killing a person. Surely, by being injected with the fluid, that kitten could have become a person, but that counterfactual is still not enough to assert that killing the kitten is as bad as killing a person. As Tolley concludes, "if it is not seriously wrong to destroy an injected kitten which will naturally develop the properties that bestow a right to life, neither can it be seriously wrong to destroy a member of Homo sapiens which lacks such properties, but will naturally come to have them" [33].

Furthermore, if potentiality for personhood is the criterion for moral status and rights, then other entities with similar potential should also be considered. For example, gametes (sperm and egg cells) also possess the potential to contribute to the creation of a new human life, yet they are not typically accorded the same moral consideration as embryos or fetuses. In fact, with the development of cloning technology, *any* human cell is now potentially a human. Does that imply that we should take extra care in handling any form of human tissue, since those entities also have moral status, given their potentiality?

Yet, a hard pill to swallow is that, if the fetus cannot be considered a person, on what grounds can a newly born child be considered a person? After all, the newly born does not have the mental attributes upon which the notion of personhood is built. If that is the case, then does that imply that, very much as abortion, infanticide may not be necessarily immoral? We have already alluded to the views of Peter Singer and Michael Tooley, for whom, in some circumstances, infanticide is ethically acceptable.

But upholders of the pro-choice view do not need to go that far. As opposed to abortion, infanticide may be immoral for other reasons, even while admitting that newly born infants are not persons. Warren attempts to establish some relevant differences. For example, she states that "if the newborn's parents do not want it, or are unable to care for it, there are (in most cases) people who are able and eager to adopt it and to provide a good home for it." Recall that in the pro-life camp, a popular slogan is "Adoption is an option." I have already explained why this slogan is problematic in the case of abortion, but it is not as problematic in the case of infanticide. After all, in that case, the child is already born, and giving it up for adoption does not require the sacrifice that is indeed required during pregnancy.

Warren acknowledges that while newly born children are not yet persons, they come very close to that status, and therefore, it would be immoral to simply kill them. Yet isn't that the case with the fetus in an advanced state of gestation? On this point, Warren argues on similar grounds as Thomson: "once the infant is born, its continued life cannot (except, perhaps, in very exceptional cases) pose any serious threat to the woman's life or health, since she is free to put it up for adoption, or, where this is impossible, to place it in a state-supported institution… In contrast, a pregnant woman's right to protect her own life and health clearly outweighs other people's desire that the fetus be preserved."

While this argument does carry some force, many people find it difficult to accept the moral permissibility of late abortions, even while admitting the moral permissibility of early abortions. If no firm moral criterion is found to distinguish both types of abortion, then clearly some cognitive dissonance is at play amongst those people. In any case, late term abortions are very rare. The focus of the debate is usually on early abortion, and on that, the moral landscape is much clearer, with pro-choice arguments carrying more force, although the debate ought to continue.

# References

1. Hull NE, Hoffer PC. Roe v. Wade: the abortion rights controversy in American history. University Press of Kansas; 2021.
2. Faux M. Roe v. Wade: the untold story of the landmark Supreme Court decision that made abortion legal. Cooper Square Press; 2000.
3. Beck R. Self-conscious dicta: the origins of Roe v. Wade's trimester framework. Am J Legal Hist. 2011;51:505.
4. Blumenthal K. Jane against the world: Roe V. Wade and the fight for reproductive rights. Roaring Brook Press; 2020.
5. Ziegler M. After Roe: the lost history of the abortion debate. Harvard University Press; 2015.
6. Balogun JA, Okonofua FE. The politics of abortion rights in the 2022 United States midterm election: lessons for fledgling democracies around the world. Afr J Reprod Health. 2023;27:9–25.
7. Newmyer RK. Norma McCorvey. 100 Americans making constitutional history: a biographical history. 2004;130.
8. US Catholic Church. Catechism of the Catholic Church. Image; 2003.
9. O'Brien GD. The Church and abortion: a catholic dissent. Rowman & Littlefield; 2023.
10. Castuera I. A social history of Christian thought on abortion: ambiguity versus certainty in moral debate. Am J Econ Soc 2017;76:121–227.
11. Noonan JT Jr. Abortion and the Catholic Church: a summary history. Nat LF. 1967;12:85.
12. Miller P. Good Catholics: the battle over abortion in the Catholic Church. University of California Press; 2014.
13. Dombrowski DA, Deltete RJ. A brief, liberal, Catholic defense of abortion. University of Illinois Press; 2000.
14. McDonagh E. Ethical problems of abortion: 1. Theology. 1968;71:393–400.
15. Barr J. Tertullian and the unborn child: Christian and pagan attitudes in historical perspective. Routledge; 2017.
16. Mistry Z. Abortion in the early Middle Ages, c. 500–900. Boydell & Brewer; 2015.
17. Jones DA. The soul of the embryo. Continuum London; 2004.
18. Riddle JM. Eve's herbs: a history of contraception and abortion in the West. Harvard University Press; 1999.
19. Riddle JM. Contraception and abortion from the Ancient World to the Renaissance. Harvard University Press; 1992.
20. Gajdusek P. Quickening Doctrine. Common L Rev 2003;5:23.
21. Haldane J, Lee P. Aquinas on human ensoulment, abortion and the value of life. Philosophy. 2003;78:255–78.
22. Aquinas T. Summa theologica. Xist Publishing; 2015.
23. Reichberg GM. Aquinas on defensive killing: a case of double effect? Thomist Speculative Q Rev. 2005;69:341–70.
24. Jones RK, Jerman J. Abortion incidence and service availability in the United States, 2014. Perspect Sex Reprod Health. 2017;49:17–27.
25. Paul II J. Memory and identity: personal reflections. Hachette UK; 2012.
26. Juergensmeyer M. Terror in the mind of God: the global rise of religious violence. University of California Press; 2017.
27. Kershnar S. Does the pro-life worldview make sense?: abortion, hell, and violence against abortion doctors. Routledge; 2017.
28. Thomson JJ. Self-defense. Philos Public Aff. 1991;283–310.
29. Brown P. Bonhoeffer: God's conspirator in a state of exception. Springer; 2019.
30. Bader EJ, Baird-Windle P. Targets of hatred: anti-abortion terrorism. St. Martin's Press; 2015.
31. Ramsey CB. Restructuring the debate over fetal homicide laws. Ohio St LJ. 2006;67:721.
32. Mills C. Making fetal persons: fetal homicide, ultrasound, and the normative significance of birth. Philosophia. 2014;4:88–107.

33. Tooley M. Abortion and infanticide. Philos Public Aff. 1972;37–65.
34. Singer P. Practical ethics. Cambridge: Cambridge University Press; 2011.
35. Buchanan TA, Xiang AH, Page KA. Gestational diabetes mellitus: risks and management during and after pregnancy. Nat Rev Endocrinol. 2012;8:639.
36. MacKay AP, Berg CJ, Atrash HK. Pregnancy-related mortality from preeclampsia and eclampsia. Obstet Gynecol. 2001;97:533–8.
37. Miller EC, Wilczek A, Bello NA, Tom S, Wapner R, Suh Y. Pregnancy, preeclampsia and maternal aging: from epidemiology to functional genomics. Ageing Res Rev. 2022;73:101535.
38. Jansen CH, Kastelein AW, Kleinrouweler CE, Van Leeuwen E, De Jong KH, Pajkrt E, et al. Development of placental abnormalities in location and anatomy. Acta Obstet Gynecol Scand. 2020;99:983–93.
39. Sharif S, Sultana S, Waqar F, Saeed A, Sadia S. Maternal and fetal outcome of pregnancies with umbilical cord problems. J Islamic Int Med College (JIIMC). 2011;6:14–8.
40. Gonzalo-Carballes M, Ríos-Vives MÁ, Fierro EC, Azogue XG, Herrero SG, Rodríguez AE, et al. A pictorial review of postpartum complications. Radiographics. 2020;40:2117–41.
41. Oyelese Y, Ananth CV. Postpartum hemorrhage: epidemiology, risk factors, and causes. Clin Obstet Gynecol. 2010;53:147–56.
42. Malmir M, Boroojerdi NA, Masoumi SZ, Parsa P. Factors affecting postpartum infection: a systematic review. Infect Disord-Drug Targets (Formerly Current Drug Targets-Infectious Disorders). 2022;22:28–37.
43. Ghaedrahmati M, Kazemi A, Kheirabadi G, Ebrahimi A, Bahrami M. Postpartum depression risk factors: a narrative review. J Educa Health Promot 2017; 6.
44. Volokh E. Medical self-defense, prohibited experimental therapies, and payment for organs. Harv L Rev. 2006;120:1813.
45. McDonagh EL. Breaking the abortion deadlock: from choice to consent. USA: Oxford University Press; 1996.
46. Zargarian T, Sadegh Pour M, Khazaei M. Conceptual coordinates of mother life threat and risk. Ther Abortion Laws J Woman Family Stud. 2021;8:2.
47. Kulier R, Kapp N, Gülmezoglu AM, Hofmeyr GJ, Cheng L, Campana A. Medical methods for first trimester abortion. Cochrane Database Syst Rev. 2011.
48. Coleman SS GD. Direct and indirect abortion in the Roman Catholic tradition: a review of the Phoenix case. Springer; 2013. p. 127–43.
49. Lymburner JA, Roesch R. The insanity defense: five years of research (1993–1997). Int J Law Psychiatry. 1999;22:213–40.
50. Allnutt S, Samuels A, O'driscoll C. The insanity defence: from wild beasts to M'Naghten. Australas Psychiatry. 2007;15:292–8.
51. Nozick R, Nagel T. Anarchy, state, and utopia. New York: Basic books; 1974.
52. Minorelli L, Ceolin GF. Why use a classic example? brief reflections about the criminal law teaching from plank of Carneades. Derecho Penal y Criminologia. 2022;43:169.
53. Joachim H. On the history of justification and excuse in cases of necessity. In: Kant and law. Routledge; 2017. p. 323–36.
54. Otsuka M. Killing the innocent in self-defense. Philos Public Aff. 1994;23:74–94.
55. Thomson JJ. A defense of abortion. Philos Public Aff. I. 1971.
56. Miller RA. The limits of bodily integrity: abortion, adultery, and rape legislation in comparative perspective. Routledge; 2016.
57. Bradley SE, Polis CB, Bankole A, Croft T. Global contraceptive failure rates: who is most at risk? Stud Fam Plann. 2019;50:3–24.
58. Trussell J. Contraceptive failure in the United States. Contraception. 2004;70:89–96.
59. Feldbrugge FM. Good and bad Samaritans: a comparative survey of criminal law provisions concerning failure to rescue. Am J Comp Law. 1965;14:630–57.
60. Malm HM. Bad Samaritan laws: harm, help, or hype? Law Phil. 2000;19:707.
61. Dressler J. Some brief thoughts (mostly negative) about Bad Samaritan laws. Santa Clara L Rev. 1999;40:971.

62. Fifield J. Why It's hard to punish 'Bad Samaritans' [Internet]. Stateline. 2017 [cited 2024 Apr 17]. Available from: https://stateline.org/2017/09/19/why-its-hard-to-punish-bad-samaritans/.
63. Segers S. The path toward ectogenesis: looking beyond the technical challenges. BMC Med Ethics. 2021;22:59.
64. Baron T. Moving forwards: a problem for full ectogenesis. Bioethics. 2021;35:407–13.
65. Pugh AN. Adoption is an option: a personal narrative. Long Beach: California State University; 2010.
66. Murray H, Baakdah H, Bardell T, Tulandi T. Diagnosis and treatment of ectopic pregnancy. CMAJ. 2005;173:905–12.
67. Haas JM. Moral theological analysis of direct versus indirect abortion. Linacre Q. 2017;84:248–60.
68. Bass M. Palliative care resuscitation. Wiley; 2006.
69. Černý D. The principle of double effect: a history and philosophical defense. Routledge; 2020.
70. Thomson JJ. Killing, letting die, and the trolley problem. In: Death, dying and the ending of life, vol. I and II. Routledge; 2019. p. V2_17-V2_30.
71. Hauser M, Cushman F, Young L, Kang-Xing Jin R, Mikhail J. A dissociation between moral judgments and justifications. Mind Lang. 2007;22:1–21.
72. Thomson JJ. Rights, restitution, and risk: essays, in moral theory. Harvard University Press; 1986.
73. Hauser MD, Young L, Cushman F. Reviving Rawls's linguistic analogy: operative principles and the causal structure of moral actions. In: Moral Psychology, vol 2: the cognitive science of morality: intuition and diversity. Cambridge, MA, US: Boston Review; 2008. p. 107–43.
74. Greene JD, Cushman FA, Stewart LE, Lowenberg K, Nystrom LE, Cohen JD. Pushing moral buttons: the interaction between personal force and intention in moral judgment. Cognition. 2009;111:364–71.
75. Petrinovich L, O'Neill P. Influence of wording and framing effects on moral intuitions. Ethol Sociobiol. 1996;17:145–71.
76. Musschenga AW. Moral intuitions, moral expertise and moral reasoning 1. J Philos Educ. 2009;43:597–613.
77. McMahan J. Intention, permissibility, terrorism, and war. Philos Perspect. 2009;23:345–72.
78. Waldmann MR, Dieterich JH. Throwing a bomb on a person versus throwing a person on a bomb: intervention myopia in moral intuitions. Psychol Sci. 2007;18:247–53.
79. Kamm FM. Intricate ethics: rights, responsibilities, and permissable harm. Oxford University Press; 2008.
80. Kamm FM. Harming some to save others. Philos Stud Int J Philos Anal Tradit. 1989;57:227–60.
81. Sulmasy D. Heart and soul: the case of the conjoined twins. America: The Jesuit Review [Internet]. 2000 Dec 2 [cited 2024 Apr 23]; Available from: https://www.americamagazine.org/issue/396/article/heart-and-soul.
82. Smart JJC, Williams B. Utilitarianism: for and against. Cambridge University Press; 1973.
83. Mills E. The egg and I: conception, identity, and abortion. Philos Rev. 2008;117:323–48.
84. Brown MT. The potential of the human embryo. J Med Philos. 2007;32:585–618.
85. Beckwith FJ. Defending life: a moral and legal case against abortion choice. Cambridge University Press; 2007.
86. Shannon TA, Walter JJ. The new genetic medicine: theological and ethical reflections. Rowman & Littlefield; 2003.
87. Kaczor C. The ethics of abortion: women's rights, human life, and the question of justice. Routledge; 2022.
88. Kadic AS, Kurjak A. Cognitive functions of the fetus. Ultraschall in der Medizin-Euro J Ultrasound. 2018;39:181–9.
89. Vanhatalo S, van Nieuwenhuizen O. Fetal pain? Brain Dev. 2000;22:145–50.
90. Warren MA. On the moral and legal status of abortion. The Monist. 1973;43–61.
91. Annis DB. Abortion and the potentiality principle. Southern J Philos. 1984;22:155.
92. Marquis D. An argument that abortion is wrong. Ethical Theory Anthology. 2013;400–9.

# Chapter 3
# Public Health

**Abstract** This chapter delves into the life story of Mary Mallon—aka Typhoid Mary—in order to discuss the complexities of medical decisions in the context of pandemics and the realm of public health at large. Some trolley dilemmas are presented to examine Michael Walzer's concept of "dirty hands"—i.e., the prospect of doing intrinsically immoral things so as to ultimately achieve favorable outcomes in situations of extreme emergency. Further trolley scenarios are discussed so as to assess whether numerical considerations are relevant in moral decision-making in the first place. Similarly, this chapter presents a series of trolley dilemmas that prompt reflection on the consideration of future generations and animals in moral decision-making. This discussion delves into the realms of population ethics and animal rights, exploring how these factors impact biomedical research and resource distribution in healthcare.

Long before Kevorkian and McCorvey, the American public had already had a taste of the culture wars in the case of Mary Mallon [1]. Born in 1869 in Ireland, Mallon immigrated to the United States in the late 19th century, like many Irish immigrants seeking better opportunities amid economic hardship and famine in Ireland. She settled in New York City, where she found work as a cook for affluent families.

Though seemingly healthy herself, Mallon was a carrier of *Salmonella typhi*, the bacterium responsible for causing typhoid fever. As a cook, she unwittingly spread the disease to multiple households where she worked. Typhoid fever is transmitted through contaminated food or water, and Mary's lack of proper hygiene, such as handwashing, contributed to the spread of the disease.

In 1906, a typhoid fever outbreak occurred in a household where Mary worked as a cook. Investigating the outbreak, public health officials traced several cases of typhoid fever to residences where Mary had been employed. This led to her identification as an asymptomatic carrier of the disease [2].

She vehemently denied being responsible for spreading typhoid fever and resisted efforts to have her quarantined. However, authorities deemed her a threat to public health and forcibly isolated her. In 1907, she was confined to North Brother Island, a quarantine facility in New York City, where she remained for three years. After

G. Andrade, *Trolleyology in Medicine*, SpringerBriefs in Ethics,
https://doi.org/10.1007/978-3-031-72806-8_3

her release from quarantine in 1910, Mallon promised to no longer work as a cook and to take precautions to prevent the spread of typhoid fever. However, she later resumed working as a cook under various aliases to evade detection. Despite her best efforts, additional typhoid fever outbreaks occurred in households where she worked, leading to further scrutiny. In 1915, Mallon was apprehended again and returned to quarantine, where she remained until her death in 1938. Throughout her life, she maintained her innocence and protested against her treatment by public health authorities.

Commentators of this case have pointed out the racial undertones [3]. The case happened during a period of heightened nativism and anti-immigrant sentiment in the United States. Anti-Irish sentiment was prevalent, fueled by stereotypes portraying the Irish as dirty, unhygienic, and disease prone. The Irish, along with other immigrant groups, were often scapegoated for various social problems, including public health crises. Mary's case thus reflected broader societal anxieties about immigration and its perceived impact on public health and social stability.

The media coverage of Mary Mallon's case often emphasized her Irish ethnicity, portraying her as a foreign threat to public health. Newspapers sensationalized her story, using inflammatory language and imagery that played into existing stereotypes about the Irish. Class was also at stake. Her socioeconomic status as a working-class immigrant further intersected with her ethnicity to shape public perceptions of her case [4]. While her case was primarily framed by the media in terms of public health concerns, her ethnicity and social class contributed to perceptions of her as a threat to societal order.

As the COVID-19 pandemic began in 2020, the case of "Typhoid Mary" was brought to the fore once again [5]. Memories of her case served as a platform to discuss the challenges of balancing individual liberties with the need to protect public health, particularly in cases involving asymptomatic carriers. Very much as with the COVID-19 pandemic, at the heart of Mary's case was the tension between protecting public health and respecting individual rights.

This issue is as relevant as ever and is a central point of contention in the culture wars. The experience with the COVID-19 pandemic has put to test many of our ethical intuitions. We still have unresolved questions: How far should vaccine mandates, mask mandates, and lockdowns go? How should we distribute medical resources in times of emergency? Trolley scenarios can shed light on some of these.

## The Problem of Dirty Hands

During the COVID-19 pandemic, governments throughout the world put in force lockdowns [6]. This is a standard procedure in public health management, as lockdowns serve various purposes. By limiting people's movement and interactions, lockdowns aim to reduce the rate at which the virus spreads from person to person.

In order to be effective, lockdowns need to be enforced by governments. Consequently, during the COVID-19 pandemic, many individuals faced sanctions (fines, imprisonment, etc.) for not complying with the rules and regulations.

North Korea went to extremes in this regard. As per some reports, one patient who did not fully comply with the strict quarantine imposed by the government "was arrested by officers and immediately shot as the country [took] sickening measures to avoid the killer outbreak spreading" [7]. This prompted the concern and protests of many institutions worldwide, as most people understand that while in times of pandemic some drastic measures ought to inevitably be taken, killing someone for violating quarantine is going too far.

The case could be made that those who violate quarantines become aggressors, and as per the principles discussed in the previous chapter, there is legitimacy to act in self-defense. Of course, the threat posed by a violator of a quarantine (even if carrying a deadly virus) is not as imminent as the ones presented in the trolley dilemmas I have discussed, so the proportional response is not to kill them in self-defense, but rather, to try to neutralize them first via other means.

But suppose the virus at stake is so contagious and deadly, that the North Korean government officials reason along the following lines: "person X is the sole carrier of this virus and she has been placed under quarantine. We will watch her movements, but we cannot be absolutely sure that she will not try to escape. If she does escape, she will spread the virus and half of our country's population will die. Even if she fully complies with the quarantine, the virus might still somehow make it to the rest of the population. It is better to kill her now. If we do so, we will save our country from a major catastrophe. We want the best for our citizens, and if that implies we need to kill her as the means to provide happiness to our country, so be it."

Most people would recoil at this idea, for the very same reasons most people choose not to push the fat man from the footbridge in order to stop the incoming trolley bound to kill five people. As discussed above, we are not really sure why we must not push the fat man (perhaps it is on account of rights, or of the doctrine of double or triple effect, etc.), but we know that it is simply not acceptable to do so.

But what if the trolley is bound to kill, not five, but ten people? What about one thousand? Or one million? Or one billion? Must we follow the Latin dictum, *Fiat iustitia ruat cælum* (Let justice be done though the heavens fall)? Or is there some point at which we might agree that the fat man must be inevitably pushed? Is it ever permissible for public health officials—especially in the context of pandemics—to get their hands dirty in doing some morally questionable work that ultimately serves the purpose of saving a huge number of lives?

This is not solely about killing people—although that certainly may be part of it—, but about doing seemingly immoral things in the context of emergencies. For example, in emergency situations, doctors may consider using experimental or unproven treatments if conventional options are unavailable or ineffective; this obviously raises ethical concerns about informed consent and the potential risks and benefits of the treatment, since the principle of informed consent is a cornerstone of medical ethics. While these actions are unconventional or morally questionable in normal circumstances, would they be justified in emergency situations?

Ethicists have discussed this possibility under the principle of "dirty hands." If the trolley were bound to kill one million people tied to the tracks, and a person decides to push the fat man from the footbridge, that act may itself be an instance of "dirty hands."

The idea that people sometimes believe they have valid reasons to engage in actions that might be considered morally wrong in the service of a larger or noble goal has long been a topic of philosophical and ethical debate. This notion is encapsulated by the writings of Niccolò Machiavelli, who famously asserted that "although the act condemns the doer, the end may justify him" [8]. Machiavelli's thoughts have often been misinterpreted or deliberately misquoted, leading to a skewed understanding of his ideas. As a result, in modern parlance, the term 'Machiavellian' has come to be associated with unscrupulous manipulation, deceit, and a willingness to do whatever it takes, regardless of ethical considerations, to achieve one's goals.

Nevertheless, Machiavelli's insights extend far beyond the simplistic view of him as a proponent of cold-blooded pragmatism. His ideas have deeply influenced modern ethical discussions, particularly in the realm of political ethics. One notable thinker who has grappled with these complex themes is Michael Walzer, who introduced the concept of "dirty hands" in political morality. Walzer's arguments primarily address the ethical dilemmas faced by politicians, though they hold relevance for other fields, including medical ethics.

Walzer contends that political leaders, who are tasked with making decisions that serve the greater good of society, often find themselves in situations where morally dubious actions might be necessary to achieve beneficial outcomes. He acknowledges the harsh reality encapsulated in the claim that "no one succeeds in politics without getting his hands dirty," [9] but he refrains from unequivocally embracing this notion. Instead, Walzer posits that there are circumstances where it is morally defensible to strive for success, even if it means compromising one's ethical purity: "sometimes it is right to try to succeed, and then it must also be right to get one's hands dirty" [9].

However, Walzer approaches this dilemma with a nuanced prudence, avoiding Machiavelli's more straightforward endorsement of immoral actions justified by their results. He aligns more closely with the philosophical stance of Albert Camus, particularly as evidenced in Camus' play *The Just Assassins*. In this work, Camus explores the moral complexities faced by individuals who resort to violence to overthrow a tyrant. The play underscores that while such drastic measures might bring about positive change, those who take such actions must also grapple with the moral weight of their deeds and accept responsibility for them.

Walzer's exploration of political ethics delves deeply into the moral predicaments that can arise in dire situations. He posits that politicians might, at times, find themselves forced into actions that conflict with their moral principles. These actions, however necessary they may seem, should never be sources of pride. Instead, they should be accompanied by a profound sense of guilt and moral conflict. Walzer argues that ethical individuals, even those holding public office, should adhere to moral rules with a strong sense of duty, viewing them as more than mere guidelines. An ordinary moral person would feel remorse when violating these rules, as this guilt is a testament to their moral integrity. Without this sense of guilt, their goodness could be called into question.

To illustrate his point, Walzer presents a scenario that has since become emblematic in discussions of ethical dilemmas. Imagine a newly elected leader who has begun negotiating with insurgents in a country under siege by terrorists. As the leader steps into office, they are confronted with a horrific choice: authorize the torture of a captured insurgent who likely possesses critical information about bombs hidden in various apartment buildings throughout the city. These bombs are set to detonate within the next twenty-four hours. Despite harboring a vehement opposition to torture, viewing it as inherently evil in any circumstance, the leader gives the authorization under the belief that it is necessary to save countless lives.

This hypothetical yet poignant example underscores Walzer's contention that the politician, while engaging in an ethically reprehensible act, is nonetheless driven by an imperative to prevent greater harm. This dilemma places the leader in an excruciating position where the choice made, although potentially the correct one under the grim circumstances, must carry the burden of guilt.

These ethical dilemmas resonate particularly in light of the surge in moral conversations following the terrorist attacks on September 11th, 2001. In their aftermath, the US government faced its own moral quandaries regarding the use of enhanced interrogation techniques, including torture, to thwart future threats. Similarly, physicians have grappled with decisions about experimental treatments and life-saving measures in emergencies. Walzer's discussion of these 'ticking bomb' situations thus catalyzes ongoing debates about the ethical boundaries of state action, as well as medical practice in the face of imminent danger, reflecting a broader struggle to reconcile the need for security and health with adherence to unwavering moral principles.

This "dirty hands" approach is obviously at odds with the doctrine of double effect. In such situations, individuals may knowingly engage in actions that conflict with their moral principles or values (e.g., not deliberately doing harm in order to bring about a greater good), with the recognition that there may be no morally pure or ideal solution to the dilemma they face.

Of course, the "dirty hands" approach to morality can be exceedingly problematic across various fields, including both political and medical ethics. The inherent issue lies in the potential for a slippery slope effect, where the initial acceptance of morally dubious actions could pave the way for increasingly unethical behavior. While Walzer cautions that his argument should be handled with great care, the numerous abuses witnessed during the "war on terror" exemplify how justifications for torture and other heinous acts can lead to a dangerous escalation. Once such rationalizations are accepted, politicians may feel emboldened to use the dirty hands approach to legitimize a wide array of abuses.

In the medical field, similar concerns arise, as physicians often confront excruciating decisions that test the boundaries of ethical practice. For instance, consider a situation where doctors must decide whether to perform high-risk experiments on patients in order to advance medical knowledge of a very common and lethal disease. In such cases, doctors may initially rationalize these actions as necessary for the greater good. However, without stringent ethical oversight and grounding, this initial acceptance of performing potentially harmful procedures could become normalized, thereby compromising the overall integrity of medical ethics. If this slippery slope is not carefully managed, the medical profession risks eroding public trust and undermining the foundational principle of "do no harm."

Allowing for immoral actions under the guise of pursuing morality itself risks breeding cynicism in both fields. In politics, if leaders frequently resort to morally questionable actions and justify them through the dirty hands approach, public trust erodes, and a culture of cynicism and skepticism takes root. Similarly, in medicine, if doctors often bypass ethical guidelines claiming necessity, it could lead to diminished trust in the healthcare system and foster a sense of futility and loss of moral direction among medical professionals.

As C. A. J. Coady aptly elucidates in his critique of Walzer, individuals can be corrupted by involvement in morally dubious actions, even when motivated by noble intentions [10]. As per this critique, the capacity for moral imagination is crucial, and Walzer's argument undermines this capacity, as the approach of accepting morally dubious actions without question is too unchanging. Coady's view suggests that before rushing to commit an unethical act—even if the ultimate goal is morally worthy—, it is imperative to undertake additional intellectual efforts to explore alternative solutions that could help in avoiding the proposed immoral action.

Furthermore, the prolonged contemplation of such moral quandaries can also lead to corruption, permeating the wider intellectual discourse and corroding the ethical fabric of society. Many of the biggest ethical breaches in the history of medicine have been motivated by noble intentions to some extent. Consider the infamous Tuskegee syphilis experiment, in which African American men were used as experimental subjects in the treatment of syphilis without their consent [11, 12]. Those who carried out this experiment argued that the study would contribute to understanding the natural progression of syphilis in untreated individuals, thereby potentially improving public health interventions. They might have convinced themselves that the potential scientific insights gained from the study justified the unethical means used to obtain them. However, this rationale demonstrated a significant lack of moral imagination. Instead of seeking ethical alternatives, the researchers chose a path that violated fundamental human rights. This infamous experiment not only failed to achieve its goals but also severely damaged public health efforts and exacerbated racial tensions in the United States.

Coady's point about the need to work towards moral imagination and find creative ways to solve problems without engaging in immoral acts is taken. But would there not be a point at which the numbers are so large that perhaps the harm towards someone is justified in serving the greater good? Pandemics have great potential to be an existential threat to humanity, so, shouldn't we consider that, in cases of extreme emergency, if it comes down to having to do some injustice to innocent people in order to save a much greater number, we must do it? Again, if the trolley is bound to kill one million people tied on the tracks, is it still not morally acceptable to push the fat man?

The normative theory of utilitarianism suggests the best action is the one that maximizes utility, or overall happiness or well-being, for the greatest number of people. Critics often highlight a perceived flaw in utilitarianism, suggesting it leads to scapegoating—killing an innocent person to save many people—[13], not unlike throwing the fat man from the bridge.

However, this argument is not necessarily conclusive. Some modifications can be made to the utilitarian doctrine in order to avoid this conclusion. For example, a proponent of rule utilitarianism might argue that sacrificing an innocent individual to placate a hostile mob would ultimately result in greater harm over time [14]. Such an act could erode trust in judicial systems, potentially leading to societal collapse, with consequences far more severe than if the innocent person had not been sacrificed. Likewise, throwing the fat man from the footbridge to save five would induce a sense of fear and uncertainty amongst common people (anybody walking on a bridge may wonder if they will be the next person to be thrown) that may easily lead to violence and the deaths of more people, thus defeating the original purpose. So, even under utilitarian considerations, it would not be morally acceptable to throw the fat man from the bridge.

Some utilitarian philosophers have bitten the bullet and have come to conclude that in the extremely unlikely scenario in which sacrificing one innocent person for the common good would actually increase utility, then such an option ought to be followed. For example, when the utilitarian philosopher J. J. C. Smart was confronted with the case of an innocent man who is framed in order to appease a mob, he responded: "surely if it is shown that, in certain circumstances (which we may hope will never in fact occur) a utilitarian ought, on his own principles, to commit a serious injustice, such as punishing an innocent man, then it seems that this does and should weaken the appeal of utilitarianism. And yet one can be made to vacillate back again. We also reflect that the serious injustice would *ex hypothesi* be the only possible alternative to an even greater total misery than would be caused by the injustice… if a case really did arise in which injustice was the lesser of two evils (in terms of human happiness and misery, that is) the anti-utilitarian conclusion is a very unpalatable one too, namely that in some circumstances one should choose the greater total misery" [15].

It is very unlikely that in the context of medical practice, there would truly come a scenario in which, as Smart phrases it, injustice was the lesser of the two evils. But if such a scenario ever comes to happen, it would probably be in the context of pandemics. The COVID-19 experience ought to teach us to be better prepared to face the challenges of pandemics, as surely, new outbreaks are bound to happen. Yet, this preparation also ought to include a moral dimension. In the context of huge numbers of victims to infectious disease, we must be prepared to consider if it is ever morally acceptable to get our hands dirty.

Walzer discussed the example of torturing a terrorist in order to avoid a nuclear blast. Likewise, we must begin to contemplate that it is at least theoretically possible to do something intrinsically horrible to avoid the spread of a deadly virus with enormous potential for harm. Walzer's example has been criticized as very unrealistic. One should hope that the scenario of having the necessity to kill some innocent person in order to prevent a pandemic is also very unrealistic. But it is important not to hastily dismiss such possibilities. It is much better to consider it as an extremely remote possibility—yet possible nevertheless—, and on that basis, decide what moral principles ought to prevail if the moment comes: doing justice even if the heavens fall, or allowing some remarkable exception to achieve a greater good? Be it as it may, it is crucial to still employ moral imagination to explore all possible ethical alternatives before resorting to extreme measures.

## Should the Numbers Count?

In the previous section, I have raised the hypothetical scenario of pushing the fat man, not just to save five persons, but a billion. If the numbers are so large, perhaps there is a point at which conventional moral principles do not apply.

But this raises another question: should numbers even matter? In Foot's original trolley scenario, the dilemma is between killing one and killing five. In that case, Foot agreed it is better to kill one, and most people—including many staunch critics of utilitarianism—would agree. We may discuss whether there are some moral principles that are beyond numbers, but *ceteris paribus*, there is an understanding that when actions follow the same pattern (i.e., comparing killing with killing, letting die with letting die, etc.), numbers do count.

This is especially the case in pandemics. In any pandemic, there's a limited availability of resources such as hospital beds, ventilators, medical personnel, and even basic supplies like masks and gloves. Numbers help policymakers and healthcare professionals make informed decisions about where to allocate these resources [16]. Ethically, this means trying to save as many lives as possible with the resources available.

But some philosophers have made the claim that in such dilemmas, the numbers should not count. As per this view, when the driver in Foot's original trolley scenario must decide whether to kill five or to kill one, no resolute decision ought to be made. At most, it should be left to chance.

The philosopher most associated with this view is John Taurek. To illustrate his views, he presents a scenario which, not unlike pandemics, concerns the allocation of medical resources. He imagines it as follows: "The situation is that I have a supply of some life-saving drug. Six people will certainly die if they are not treated with the drug. But one of the six requires all of the drug if he is to survive. Each of the other five requires one fifth of the drug. What ought I to do" [17]?

Taurek asserts that a coin should be flipped to decide who gets the pill, because moral decisions cannot be made on the basis of such numerical calculations. He explains: "often we must choose between bestowing benefits on certain people, or preventing certain harms from befalling them, and bestowing benefits on or preventing harms from befalling certain others. We cannot do both. The general question discussed here is whether we should, in such trade-off situations, consider the relative numbers of people involved as something in itself of significance in determining our course of action. The conclusion I reach is that we should not" [17].

Taurek's philosophical stance is grounded in the belief that each human life holds innate and incomparable worth. This intrinsic value, he argues, resists any form of aggregation or numerical moral assessment. From Taurek's viewpoint, the tragedy of losing one life carries immense weight in its own right and cannot be measured against the loss of many lives. When faced with situations where more than one person dies, the grief experienced does not escalate simply due to the increased number of individuals; the sorrow is profound and unwavering whether it pertains to a single life or several. As Taurek explains: "each person's potential loss has the same significance to me, only as a loss to that person alone. Because, by hypothesis, I have an equal concern for each person involved, I am moved to give each of them an equal chance to be spared his loss [17].

Taurek's argument is largely motivated by the fact that, in those types of situations, numbers may not be the most relevant criterion to decide whom to save. Suppose that in Foot's original dilemma, the one person tied to the track is the driver's personal friend. Would the driver still believe that it is better to save the other five instead of his own friend? We do not know. But if he said that he is not willing to kill one—his own friend—in order to save the five, should we morally condemn the driver? Taurek thinks not; we are allowed to give friends special considerations. Yet, if it is fine for the trolley driver to make an exception if the one person tied to the tracks is his friend, then the trolley driver should have considered all along that such decisions cannot be driven by numerical aspects.

Nevertheless, even if the trolley driver might chance his stance were the one person tied to the track his friend, it remains uncertain whether he was morally justified in doing so. If we condemn nepotism and discrimination, it is typically due to their inherent unfairness. The mere fact that someone is our friend should not sway our judgment regarding how to optimize resource allocation. Individuals are expected to adhere to their obligations when determining whom to prioritize, irrespective of the level of kinship or friendship involved.

The principle of impartial beneficence, championed by utilitarian philosophers, stands as a cornerstone idea in ethical thought. As articulated by Bentham, it dictates that each individual should hold equal weight in moral calculations—no one person counts for more than another [18]. This principle, central to medical ethics, underscores the importance of viewing every individual through a lens of equality, irrespective of their societal status. By adhering to impartial beneficence, the practice of distributing resources becomes rationalized and devoid of favoritism based on personal connections. In scenarios like the classic trolley problem, where difficult moral choices must be made, recognizing the equal value of every human life becomes paramount. In this framework, distinctions such as social standing or personal relationships should hold no bearing on the evaluation of interests; rather, each person's welfare must be assessed on a level playing field.

Taurek's argument seems to imply that, when considering whether to kill one or five in the trolley dilemma, leaving the decision to chance is actually the egalitarian approach. As per this argument, each person should be given the same chance to survive; on the basis of a coin flip, the one person on the track has a 50% chance of being rescued, and each of the other five persons on the other track have a 50% chance of being rescued.

Yet, instead of tallying the likelihood of survival for each individual, we ought to consider the inherent value of each person. If, as Bentham posits, each individual is to be considered as equal to one another, then it logically follows to prioritize saving the five over the one. This approach aligns with true egalitarianism. Derek Parfit articulately elucidates this point: "Why do we save the larger number? Because we *do* give equal weight to saving each. Each counts for one. That is why more count for more" [19].

Certainly, the expectation to treat each individual as if they mattered only as much as one is quite rigorous. It could be argued that the bond with the person on the track, if it happens to be the driver's friend, should not sway the decision of saving one person versus five. However, many of us likely display some level of hypocrisy in this scenario. When forced to make a choice, saving a friend might take precedence over saving a larger group of strangers. This inconsistency in our actions does not necessarily invalidate the utilitarian ethical viewpoint. Rather, it highlights the need for us to strive harder to align with it.

On the other hand, we could recognize that there are varying degrees of moral significance in different actions. This notion is often referred to by ethicists as the "scala" version of utilitarianism [20]. While opting to rescue a friend instead of a considerably larger group of strangers (or even an entire nation) does not label someone as morally deplorable, those who prioritize saving the greater number could be viewed as more morally praiseworthy. Therefore, even though we can empathize with individuals who don't solely rely on numerical calculations when faced with the dilemma of saving a friend or a larger group of strangers, it does not diminish the importance of considering numbers in the ethical decision-making process.

Some may find utilitarianism overly stringent, yet critics often overlook that alternative ethical frameworks could impose even greater demands on those affected by actions left undone. Suppose it is too demanding for the trolley driver to run over his friend; thus, we deem it right for the driver to divert the trolley towards the track with five people. However, this decision leads to five dead people. Isn't this equally demanding for those who were run over by the trolley, especially considering their larger number? David Sobel adeptly articulates this argument as follows: "why is Consequentialism [i.e., utilitarianism] too demanding on the person who would suffer significant costs if he was to aid others as Consequentialism requires, but non-Consequentialist morality is not similarly too demanding on… the person who would suffer more significant costs if she were not aided as the alternative to Consequentialism permits" [21]?

Therefore, *pace* Taurek's views, in navigating ethical dilemmas, particularly those involving matters of life and death, the consideration of numbers emerges as a critical aspect, especially in contexts such as public health crises. The allocation of resources during pandemics underscores the necessity of weighing the numerical impact of actions to maximize the preservation of life. Ultimately, the ongoing dialogue surrounding the role of numbers in moral decision-making underscores the complex interplay between principles, consequences, and individual considerations.

## What Numbers Should Count?

As per the arguments presented above, we can safely assume that the numbers should count. But a much more difficult question is: what numbers? Consider this scenario: a trolley is on its way to run over five people tied to the tracks, and the driver can pull a lever to divert the trolley towards another track where one person is tied. This time, we know something about the people tied to the tracks. Those five tied to the track are each ninety years old, whereas the one tied to the other track is twenty years old. Should the driver pull the lever?

This kind of dilemma is often encountered in pandemics, as it was certainly the case during the COVID-19 pandemic [22, 23]. In that particular instance, it was established early on that the virus was likely to be far more fatal amongst those of advanced age. Older adults, especially those aged 65 and above, were more likely to experience severe complications, including pneumonia, respiratory failure, and death, if infected with COVID-19 [24, 25]. The risk increased substantially with age, with those over 85 being at the highest risk. Older adults were more likely to have underlying health conditions such as heart disease, diabetes, and respiratory issues, which further increased their vulnerability to severe illness from COVID-19. Aging is associated with a decline in immune function, making older adults less capable of mounting a robust immune response to the virus, which may have prolonged the illness and increased the likelihood of complications.

For those reasons, it was generally agreed that the elderly required special attention during the COVID-19 pandemic. But if we assume that a particular threat (either a virus, or an incoming trolley, for that matter) affects both the young and the elderly on an equal basis, who should have priority in care?

The *prima facie* point of trolley dilemmas is utilitarianism and saving the greatest number of lives. Of course, as discussed in the previous chapters, there are caveats to this rule, but *ceteris paribus*, the best option is to save the greatest number of lives. However, that is not necessarily the case in the way public health policies are designed. For, the relevant criterion may not be to save the greatest number of lives, but rather, the greatest number of years to be lived.

Suppose that in the trolley dilemma presented above, the life expectancy of all six people tied to the tracks is ninety-five. If the lever is not pulled, five ninety-year-old people would die; this would imply a loss of twenty-five years. In contrast, if the lever is pulled, one twenty-year-old person would die; this would imply the loss of seventy-five years.

Death is bad for everyone, but a case could be made that it is worse for those who are deprived of more. As per the deprivation account, death is bad because it deprives individuals of the valuable experiences, relationships, and opportunities they would have had if they had continued to live; death is considered bad because it cuts short the potential for future goods that individuals would have experienced had they lived longer [26]. This implies that, if it comes to deciding between saving a twenty-year-old person and a ninety-year-old person, it is better to save the twenty-year-old person, as that person would be deprived of more in the event of her death.

Yet, number of years saved cannot be the sole criterion either. The quality of those years surely counts as well. Suppose a trolley is on its way to run one fifty-year-old person who is extremely and chronically depressed; the driver can pull a lever to divert the trolley towards the tracks, where one person is tied to the tracks, and this person is sixty years old, and is living a happy, fulfilling life. Should the lever be pulled?

If we are concerned with saving the greatest number of years, it would probably be better to not pull the lever, as the depressed fifty-year-old person is likely to have a lower life expectancy—and may even die sooner than the other person—, given her poor quality of life. However, even assuming that both people have the same life expectancy, it may still be preferable to save the sixty-year-old person, on the grounds of the quality of the years that are saved.

This reasoning rests on the assumption that survival and quantity of time cannot be the sole variable in this type of moral decision-making. Additionally, an adequate living standard after the intervention must also be taken into account. The fusion of quantitative and qualitative elements has been integrated into the Quality-Adjusted Life-Year (QALY) metric, a widely utilized tool in the field of public health. The National Institute for Health and Care Excellence (NICE) offers the following definition of QALY: "A measure of the state of health of a person or group in which the benefits, in terms of length of life, are adjusted to reflect the quality of life. One quality-adjusted life year (QALY) is equal to 1 year of life in perfect health. QALYs are calculated by estimating the years of life remaining for a patient following a particular treatment or intervention and weighting each year with a quality-of-life score (on a 0–1 scale). It is often measured in terms of the person's ability to carry out the activities of daily life, and freedom from pain and mental disturbance" [27].

When utilized in the realm of public health policy, this method empowers decision-makers to determine the allocation of funds for various medical interventions. Alan Williams, a key figure in shaping this concept, elaborates on this concept: "the essence of QALY is that it takes a year of healthy life expectancy to be worth one, but regards a year of unhealthy life expectancy as worth less than 1... The general idea is that a beneficial health care activity is one that generates a positive amount of QALYs, and that an efficient health care activity is one where the cost of QALY is as low as it can be. A high priority health care activity is one where the cost-per-QALY is low, and a low priority activity is one where cost-per-QALY is high" [28].

The notion in question may initially come across as logical and straightforward; however, it harbors a nuanced and intricate layer of QALY that often evades full acknowledgment. QALY, beyond its role in informing treatment choices, plays a pivotal role in directing which segments of the population are deemed deserving of medical interventions. Through its lens of efficiency, QALY might dictate that specific individuals grappling with particular illnesses (or, in more alarming scenarios, those belonging to certain demographic cohorts) should be excluded from receiving treatment. This exclusionary stance arises from the perception that providing treatment to such individuals may yield minimal benefits in terms of recovery or prolonged lifespan. This delineation sets the stage for biased practices and potential discrimination to seep into healthcare decision-making processes.

In this intricate web of healthcare ethics and societal dynamics, QALY poses a significant risk of eroding the foundational principle of equality that underpins truly democratic societies. In the democratic ethos, it becomes paramount to abstain from conferring preferential treatment based on inherent characteristics like race, gender, or sexual orientation. While QALY itself may not actively engage in discriminatory practices, its subtle influence can inadvertently perpetuate existing disparities, leading to a scenario where already privileged groups with longer life expectancies (often a byproduct of societal circumstances) gain further advantages in healthcare access and quality of life. This situation leaves marginalized individuals, who have historically borne the brunt of societal injustices, grappling with reduced quality of life and limited healthcare options. Consequently, as a compounding effect of this systemic injustice, they face a secondary form of discrimination within healthcare systems, all in the name of streamlining and maximizing efficiency.

Several commentators have observed the instances of double jeopardy associated with QALYs [29–31]. John Harris examines the scenario of an individual who has experienced an accident: "QALYs dictate that because an individual is unfortunate, because she has once become a victim of disaster, we are required to visit upon her a second and perhaps graver misfortune. The first disaster leaves her with a poor quality of life and QALYs then require that in virtue of this she be ruled out as a candidate for lifesaving treatment, or at best, that she be given little or no chance of benefiting from what little amelioration her condition admits of. Her first disaster leaves her with a poor quality of life and when she presents herself for help, along come QALYs and finish her off!" [32].

Another problem that must be assessed in considering the adequacy of QALYs is whether interpersonal aggregation is morally acceptable. Let us return to the trolley scenario presented at the beginning of this section: our dilemma is to save either one twenty-year-old person, or five ninety-year-old persons. The QALY approach would entail saving the former, as more years are saved. This would imply counting the number of years across various persons. We have already established that the numbers should count, but in doing so, should we aggregate interpersonally?

Critics of utilitarianism have long opposed this approach, as it does not seem to take sufficiently into account the separateness of persons [33–35]. As per this view, utilitarianism might justify actions that sacrifice the interests or rights of individuals for the greater good, since in the grand scheme of things, utility is maximized. As John Rawls famously explained, "[utilitarianism] is the consequence of extending to society the principle of choice for one man, and then, to make this extension work, conflating all persons into one… Utilitarianism does not take seriously the distinction between persons" [36].

In utilitarian calculations, the well-being or preferences of different individuals can be combined or aggregated to determine the overall utility of a situation. This means that the happiness or suffering of one person can be weighed against the happiness or suffering of another, with no inherent qualitative difference between them.

This approach may be problematic to the extent that it overlooks the moral significance of individual persons and their inherent worth. In aggregating interpersonally, persons are assumed to be containers of units that are simply added up, rather than distinct and valuable beings with their own rights and autonomy.

The problem with interpersonal aggregation becomes even more salient when we contrast a large harm done to one person, with small harms done to many persons. Consider this dilemma presented by Eliezer Yudkowsky: "Would you prefer that one person be horribly tortured for fifty years without hope or rest, or that $3^{\wedge\wedge\wedge}3$ people get dust specks in their eyes" [37]?

It is important to keep in perspective the size of the number $3^{\wedge\wedge\wedge}3$. Yudkowsky explains it as follows: "$3^{\wedge\wedge\wedge}3$ is an exponential tower of 3s which is 7,625,597,484,987 layers tall. You start with 1; raise 3 to the power of 1 to get 3; raise 3 to the power of 3 to get 27; raise 3 to the power of 27 to get 7,625,597,484,987; raise 3 to the power of 7,625,597,484,987 to get a number much larger than the number of atoms in the universe, but which could still be written down in base 10, on 100 square kilometers of paper; then raise 3 to that power; and continue until you've exponentiated 7,625,597,484,987 times. That's $3^{\wedge\wedge\wedge}3$" [37]. Yudkowsky goes on to argue that upon adding the utility value of $3^{\wedge\wedge\wedge}3$ persons, it turns out that it is better to torture one person than to allow that huge number of people to have dust specks.

This type of strict utilitarian reasoning seems very counterintuitive. For example, T. M. Scanlon presents the following scenario: "Suppose that Jones has suffered an accident in the transmitter room of a television station. Electrical equipment has fallen on his arm, and we cannot rescue him without turning off the transmitter for fifteen minutes. A World Cup match is in progress, watched by many people, and it will not be over for an hour. Jones's injury will not get any worse if we wait, but his hand has been mashed and he is receiving extremely painful electrical shocks. Should we rescue him now or wait until the match is over? Does the right thing to do depend on how many people are watching—whether it is one million or five million or a hundred million" [38]?

Intuitions indicate that even if millions of people would be deprived of the pleasure of watching a World Cup game, that is no match for the suffering the one person is undergoing by receiving extremely painful shocks. Therefore, there is a moral imperative to interrupt the transmission of the game. The numbers should count, but when the harms to different persons are unequal, we cannot simply aggregate them and decide on that basis.

This insight is especially relevant in the context of pandemics. As lockdowns became common in order to curb the spread of the COVID-19 virus, some people raised objections on economic grounds [39, 40]. As per their reasoning, lockdowns often forced many businesses to close temporarily or even permanently, leading to job losses, reduced incomes, and economic hardship for individuals and families. Likewise, lockdowns were believed to lead to a significant contraction in economic activity, as consumer spending, investment, and production were curtailed. Ulti-mately, some critics argued that the economic costs of lockdowns outweighed their potential benefits in terms of reducing COVID-19 transmission and saving lives [41].

This type of reasoning relied on interpersonal aggregation. Saving a few lives came at the expense of the small sufferings of a much larger number of people. Ultimately, the argument could be made that removing lockdowns added up utility more efficiently. After all, economic hardship does translate into quality of living. The whole point of interpersonal aggregative reasoning is that adding small grievances from a very large number of people can outweigh the large suffering of a single person.

Yet, in thinking along those lines, some essential ethical principle seems lost. Frances Kamm explains it as follows: "in translating economic loss into life years lost, we must not lose sight of the fact that if 40 million people each lose one year of life no one of those people will suffer a loss as great as someone who, for example, dies at the age of forty, thereby losing thirty years of life... There is no one person who suffers the loss of 40 million years of life and there may be no one in the large group who dies at 40 rather than 70" [42]. Ultimately, it seems we must follow some form of pairwise comparison so as to enact moral principles. In order for numbers to be counted, harms must be compared with similar harms. In Foot's original trolley scenario, there is no objection to diverting the trolley to kill one instead of killing five, because ultimately, they would all suffer the same harm, i.e., death. In that situation, it makes moral sense to engage in moral mathematics. But when the harms are not comparable (e.g., torture vs. dust specks), it seems that it is not morally adequate to simply add units of pleasure.

Nevertheless, there are some indications that there may be some breaking point at which interpersonal aggregation is indeed morally warranted. Suppose a trolley is on its way to run over one hundred people whose lower part of their bodies are tied to the tracks; if they are run over by the trolley, their legs will be amputated and they will survive, although they will have very difficult lives with considerable pain. The driver can divert the trolley towards the track where one person is tied, and upon being run over, will die. Should the trolley be diverted? Certainly, the harm of death is not comparable to the harm of having both legs amputated and having a difficult and painful life. But presumably, to many people (again, this is a matter that needs to be tested empirically), there is justification in diverting the trolley.

Indeed, some philosophers have gone farther in upholding interpersonal aggre-gation even for smaller harms in the context of public health. Consider speed limits [43]. It is well-established that speed limits save lives in various ways [44, 45]. Driving within the speed limit helps to maintain control of the vehicle and reduces the likelihood of accidents caused by excessive speed. Likewise, higher speeds result in greater kinetic energy, which translates into more forceful collisions in the event of an accident; by enforcing speed limits, authorities aim to reduce the severity of accidents and mitigate the risk of serious injuries or fatalities.

But placing the speed limit too low is massively inconvenient for the practicalities of life in industrial society. Surely some lives would be saved, but at the expense of the unhappiness of a large number of people. The harms cannot be properly compared, as dying in a car accident is a much greater harm than doubling the time to get to work. But it does seem that most people agree that speed limits can only go so far. A speed limit of, say, 20 km/h on highways would save more lives, but no government is willing to implement it.

In fact, we reason along those lines on a constant basis. We consider rational going to the pharmacy to get some relief for a minor headache, even if going there, there is still a very small chance that we might get killed by a car. Are we willing to endure the headache in order to reduce the risk of being killed by a car on our way to the pharmacy? In those cases, again, the harms cannot be compared: being run over by a car is far worse than a headache, yet we are still prepared to claim that the presentness of the headache outweighs the probability of being run over by the car.

In light of this, Alaistair Norcross explains: "many philosophers claim that certain great harms, such as death, cannot be outweighed by any number of small benefits, such as relief from headaches. And yet these same philosophers not only incur the risk of such large harms in pursuit of the small benefits, but claim that it is rational to do so. There is, at the very least, a tension between these claims, and perhaps an outright inconsistency. Of course, it's not only philosophers who willingly and knowingly accept small risks of great harms for the sake of small benefits. The vast majority of people do so" [46].

In examining the ethical complexities surrounding the prioritization of lives—particularly in scenarios akin to the classic trolley problem as applied to pandemics and public health at large—this discussion reveals the intricate interplay between quantity and quality of life, as well as the inherent challenges of interpersonal aggregation. While utilitarian principles suggest that the numbers should count, and indeed, in some instances, they seemingly do, such as diverting a trolley to save the lives of many over one, the application of this principle encounters significant moral quandaries when the harms to individuals are not directly comparable. Ultimately, the ethical calculus in such dilemmas demands a nuanced consideration of both quantitative and qualitative factors. As we navigate complex moral landscapes, it is essential to confront these ethical tensions by recognizing that while numbers may inform decisions, there may be some moral cases that are beyond quantitative considerations.

## Should Future People Count?

We have discussed the intricacies of moral decision-making when different harms are compared. A similar complication arises when different persons are compared. Do present people have the same moral worth as future people? In the previous chapter, we discussed some persuasive arguments purporting to show that even if an embryo is potentially a person, it does not have the same rights as an actual person. The embryo will be person in the future, but it does not have rights at present. Furthermore, we acknowledged that in a trolley dilemma it is intuitive to rescue one person over five embryos in petri dishes.

But now some reconsideration is needed. Perhaps there is some moral status in potentiality to the extent that future people are also relevant in moral calculations. Think about this situation: a trolley is on its way to run over one person tied to the track, and the trolley can be diverted to other tracks where nobody is present; however, if the trolley is diverted, it will activate a mechanism that will kill five persons one hundred years from now. Should the trolley be diverted?

It seems strange to think that somehow our actions are less harmful if their impact is materialized far into the future. Some people might think that, to the extent that we are chronologically closer to the person currently tied to the tracks, we have more obligations towards her. But why should that be the case?

Many philosophers would argue that geographical proximity is not a powerful criterion in moral decision-making [47–49]. Consider this scenario: a trolley is heading towards one person tied to the track, but it can be diverted towards another track where it will continue for 10,000 km, and then it will run over five persons tied to the tracks; should the trolley be diverted? It would seem strange to prefer to save one person over five, simply because those five are farther away.

Indeed, in a famous thought experiment, Peter Singer posits that if you pass by a pond and have the moral duty to rescue a drowning child, you have the same moral obligation to rescue dying children located thousands of kilometers away— Singer argues that you could at least donate to charity to prevent infant mortality in developing countries [50].

But if spatial distance does not matter, then why should temporal distance matter? The harm done by the trolley running over five persons 10,000 km away from here is as bad as the harm done by the trolley running over five persons 100 years from now. Admittedly, those five persons do not yet exist, but they are still morally relevant.

Derek Parfit presents a thought experiment that seems to confirm this intuition: "Suppose that I leave some broken glass in the undergrowth of a wood. A hundred years later this glass wounds a child. My act harms this child. If I had safely buried the glass, this child would have walked through the wood unharmed. Does it make a moral difference that the child whom I harm does not now exist" [51]? No, it does not. You would be morally wrong to leave the broken glass while in full knowledge that in the future, a currently non-existent person will be harmed.

That is the whole point of caring for the environment. This is a major area of concern in public health policies [52]. Public health professionals advocate for policies that promote environmental protection, such as regulations on pollution emissions, waste management, and conservation measures; these policies help mitigate environmental risks and prevent adverse health effects from exposure to pollutants. Likewise, environmental factors, such as air and water quality, climate change, and exposure to toxins, can contribute to the spread of diseases, especially in the future. Furthermore, public health initiatives encourage sustainable behaviors that reduce environmental degradation and improve public health outcomes.

Most beneficiaries of these policies are people in the future, and such policies do come at some of our expense in the present. But again, the fact that the beneficiaries do not yet exist does not imply that we have no obligations towards them. It is only sensible to avoid environmental degradation, even if the people who will benefit the most from our current efforts will only come to exist in the future.

Now, if we accept that we do have obligations towards the future, is it not the very first obligation to bring them to existence in the first place? Wouldn't bringing more people into existence contribute to an increase in happiness? It seems clear that, in some cases, bringing new people to the world makes it worse. Consider infants born with incurable, agonizing illnesses, facing lives likely filled with brief existence and intense pain. In such instances, the consensus might lean towards the idea that adding such lives to the population would be undesirable.

However, should there not be consistency in our stance toward population growth? If adding certain lives is deemed detrimental, wouldn't it be beneficial to add individuals whose lives are deemed worth living? Certain individuals may resist acknowledging this symmetry. They argue that by bringing into existence individuals with lives deemed unworthy, we inflict harm upon them [53]. Conversely, they posit that failing to bring into existence individuals with lives deemed worthy does not cause harm, as no existing person is harmed.

This asymmetry has been famously defended by Jan Narveson, who posited that he was "in favor of making people happy, but neutral about making happy people" [54]. Narveson upholds the so-called "intuition of neutrality": as per this view, while it is bad to bring into existence people with lives not worth living, it is neutral to bring into existence people with good lives. Presumably, many people share this intuition.

However, the intuition of neutrality has been challenged by a growing number of ethicists [55, 56]. Indeed, upon deeper contemplation, it becomes evident that we cannot remain neutral regarding the inclusion of individuals whose lives we collectively agree are worth living. If neutrality were the case, the decision to have a child or not would hold no preference. However, it is undeniable that we would strongly desire the child to lead a wholly fulfilling life rather than one that is only partially satisfactory but still deemed worth living. If true neutrality existed, both outcomes (full satisfaction versus half satisfaction) would hold equal weight, as the addition of lives worth living would not inherently improve the world. Yet, our clear preference for the former option suggests that we are not neutral regarding the addition of individuals. This implies that, when it comes to population, more is indeed better [57].

This reasoning has implications for the role of medicine in facing the prospect of human extinction. An important question in this context is: should we even care about human extinction at all? Certainly, cataclysmic events such as, say, asteroid impacts or nuclear wars may make humanity go extinct, and this would be a very unfortunate prospect, since a large number of people would have painful deaths. But what if humanity simply fades out painlessly until the last human dies without descendants? Is that so bad?

Some philosophers have argued that, indeed, human extinction is not necessarily a bad prospect [58]. For example, Jonathan Schell writes as follows: "although extinction might appear to be the largest misfortune that mankind could ever suffer, it doesn't seem to happen to anybody"; [59] similarly, Elizabeth Finneron-Burns poses the question: "If there is no form of intelligent life in the future, who would there be to lament its loss" [60].

In reply, one can argue that the prospect of human extinction would be bad because even if there are no humans around to lament that state, it affects future generations and carries opportunity costs. Those generations could have come to exist, and yet did not. Furthermore, this opportunity cost is even larger when we consider that the bulk of human population throughout history is in the future. Therefore, extinction would prevent that huge number of people from coming to exist. As William MacAskill explains: "there could be very large numbers of future people. Humanity might last for a very long time. If we last as long as the typical mammalian species, it would mean there are hundreds of thousands of years ahead of us. If history were a novel, we may be living on its very first page. Barring catastrophe, the vast majority of people who will ever live have not been born yet" [61].

Now, on this basis, there may be some unexpected implications. If medicine is deeply committed to avoiding the prospect of extinction, then it may need to reorder some of its priorities. As it stands, medicine is largely concerned with the prevention and treatment of diseases that are very prevalent. Yet, even the most serious and widespread of such illnesses are unlikely to constitute a true existential threat to our species, and therefore, are not altogether relevant in the context of avoiding human extinction. In contrast, there may be as yet unknown diseases that do constitute a serious existential threat to our survival as a species.

The philosophy of "longtermism" suggests that because the number of people in the future is far higher than the number of people in the present, we ought to give priority to ensure that those future people come to exist, and that implies focusing on existential threats, even at the expense of dedicating efforts to solving public health problems—such as AIDS—that, although very serious, do not represent a threat to our survival as a species. Nick Bostrom explains this principle as follows: "But tragic as such events [AIDS and other serious shortcomings in public health] are to the people immediately affected, in the big picture of things—from the perspective of humankind as a whole—even the worst of these catastrophes are mere ripples on the surface of the great sea of life. They haven't significantly affected the total amount of human suffering or happiness or determined the long-term fate of our species" [62].

As per this reasoning, allocating resources to the management of AIDS is not as important as allocating resources to the management of some possible (but not yet present) virus that could have the real potential to wipe us out as a species. These implications are somewhat disturbing. Certainly, the prospect of human extinction is worrisome, and medical practice ought to contribute to ensuring the continuity of our species. But to neglect the relevance of the actual suffering of current people, and instead focus our priorities on the slim chance of an event that could make our species extinct, seems morally unwarranted.

Consider this scenario: a trolley is on its way to run over five people tied to the tracks, and it could be diverted to other tracks where no persons are tied, but a landmine is located. This landmine is most likely harmless, but there is an extremely small probability (say, 0.000000000000000000000000000000001) that, if activated, it could kill the entire human species. Should the driver divert the trolley? Bostrom's reasoning suggests that the trolley should not be diverted (and hence those five persons would die), because the deaths of those five people, bad as it may be for them, are not existential risks to the human species.

Yet, most people's intuitions would probably not be in line with this decision. Indeed, this evokes a problem known in philosophy as "Pascal's mugging" [63, 64]. This is a situation in which an agent encounters a highly improbable but potentially catastrophic event. Despite its low probability, the magnitude of the event's consequences is so enormous that it seems to outweigh the low probability, leading to a dilemma for decision-making. It seems that as per the basic tenets of decision theory, agents should allocate significant resources to highly unlikely events solely based on their potential outcomes. But this reasoning can eventually lead to absurd conclusions; for example, a mugger could convince you to give him your wallet with ten dollars, on the extremely unlikely (but not impossible) promise that, tomorrow, the mugger will return to you ten billion dollars. This indicates that, once again, principles in decision-making (and even more so in the moral realm) cannot be assumed mechanically, but rather, a case-by-case consideration is necessary.

Be that as it may, let us return to the issue of whether adding people to the world is morally neutral. I have already suggested that it does seem that the intuition of neutrality is not warranted, and indeed, adding people to the world is a good thing. There seems to be a moral imperative for medical practitioners to provide assistance in fertility treatments. Of course, these efforts are directed towards improving the well-being of individuals and couples who desire to have children but face challenges due to infertility; by offering these treatments, medical professionals seek to alleviate their suffering and promote the physical, emotional, and social well-being of their patients. But fertility treatments may also be ethically justified to the extent that they increase the amount of good in the world by bringing more people to exist (provided, of course, their lives are worth living).

This reasoning is not exempt from some shortcomings. If the world population is continuously expanding, that puts pressure on our resources, and ultimately, our lives would be miserable. This concern was expressed by Thomas Malthus in the 19th Century, who famously issued this warning: "The power of population is so superior to the power in the earth to produce subsistence for man, that premature death must in some shape or other visit the human race" [65].

Malthus' warnings have been disputed by many demographers, [66–68] but for the sake of reasoning let us assume that, yes, there is a point at which, if world population keeps increasing, all our lives would be miserable, even not worth living. It is precisely for this reason that public health officials and medical practitioners take very seriously the need for the availability of birth controls in many regions of the world, especially in developing countries.

But what if we were to increase population size significantly, thereby potentially reducing overall quality of life, but not to the extent that life becomes not worth living? Imagine a scenario where we have an enormous population enduring lives that are just marginally worth living. In such a situation, wouldn't an increase in population still be preferable?

This elicits a dilemma in utilitarian ethics. In this school of thought, it is agreed that utility ought to be maximized. But shall that be done on an average or aggregate basis? Consider this scenario: a trolley is on its way to run over five persons tied to the tracks who are mildly depressed, but their lives are still worth living, and each has a happiness level of 50. The driver could divert the trolley towards a track where one person is tied; this person is very happy, with happiness level 100. Should the trolley be diverted?

If the five persons are saved, 250 units of happiness would be preserved; if the one person is saved, 100 units of happiness would be preserved. However, if the five persons are saved, each of those persons would have 50 units of happiness, whereas if the one person is saved, that person would have 100 units of happiness. If we embrace total utilitarianism, we would choose to save the five, as more happiness units are preserved; if we embrace average utilitarianism, we would choose to save the one person, as more happiness units *per person* are preserved. People's responses to this particular dilemma need to be empirically tested yet, but it does seem that, in most situations, most people lean towards average utilitarianism [69].

In terms of population size, most people seem to think it is better to have a smaller world population with a higher standard of living, than a larger world population with a lower standard of living. Indeed, Derek Parfit famously described as "repugnant" the following conclusion: "For any possible population of at least ten billion people, all with a very high quality of life, there must be some much larger imaginable population whose existence, if other things are equal, would be better even though its members have lives that are barely worth living" [51]. Presumably, most people are also repugned by this prospect.

Yet, however unsettling, this conclusion possesses its own logic. In matters of happiness, it appears that the aggregate number holds greater significance than average measures, and this can be concluded on the basis of the so-called "mere addition paradox" [70–72]. Let us delve into a different scenario for better clarity. Picture yourself as an educator organizing a field trip for 20 students scheduled for Thursday. Initially, the school designates $10 for each student, summing up to $200. However, a sudden twist occurs on Tuesday as the principal revises the arrangement, including an extra 20 students; the budget for that new group will be $5 per student. Even though the additional students may not experience the same level of enjoyment as the original group, they are still anticipated to derive pleasure from the trip. This alteration leads to a total budget boost to $300. Does this modification hold merit? Indeed, it does, as it ensures the original group is not disadvantaged, accommodates the newcomers, and expands the budget.

In a twist of events, the principal, displeased with inequalities, suggests on Wednesday an equal distribution of the budget among all students, adding an extra $50 to the pool. This elevates the budget to $350, granting each student $8.75. Is this revised arrangement an improvement? Once again, the answer is affirmative, as it fosters equity compared to Tuesday's setup and enhances the overall budget. Consequently, the Wednesday proposition outshines both the Tuesday and Monday blueprints, indicating a progressive refinement over time.

In contrast to Monday's strategy, Wednesday's approach amplifies both the participant count and the total budget. Despite a dip in the average budget allocated per student from $10 to $8.75, we prioritize other aspects, deeming Wednesday's plan as the superior choice. This underscores a preference for total measures over mere averages.

Now, let us reconsider world population size. Is a population of 1 billion people, each with a happiness level of 50, preferable to a population of 100 billion people, each with a happiness level of 1 (yet still with lives deemed worthwhile)? Following the logic above, which favors total measures, 100 billion units of happiness outweigh 50 billion units. If we were to prioritize averages, adding one person with an extremely low quality of life would seem preferable to adding 1 billion people with slightly reduced happiness levels. This conclusion appears absurd and underscores the primacy of total measures.

Yet, it is still understandable that most people would be disturbed by the possibility of a very crowded world with lower standards of living. While Parfit's conclusion may have a logic of its own, it is still repugnant, and public health practitioners ought not to lightly dismiss the wisdom of repugnance in the context of population ethics as applied to issues such as distribution of fertility treatments and availability of birth control. In putting to test our intuitions, it seems that in some scenarios, most of us would accept counting future generations in our moral calculations, but in some others, that approach may lead to absurd (or at least uncomfortable) conclusions. Likewise, our intuitions about average vs. total measures of well-being may also be conflicted. Yet, trolley dilemmas (and other thought experiments) are still relevant, to the extent that they may help medical practitioners test some intuitions, in order to clarify the relevant moral principles and apply them in the context of public health ethics.

## Should Animals Count?

The COVID-19 pandemic has been managed with the development of research about the workings of the virus and the production of vaccines. In this endeavor, animal experimentation has played an important role [73–75]. Animal studies have been integral in the development and testing of COVID-19 vaccines [76, 77]. Before human clinical trials could begin, vaccines underwent rigorous testing in animal models to evaluate their safety, efficacy, and immune response. These studies provided valuable insights into vaccine candidates' ability to induce protective immunity and identify potential adverse effects.

Likewise, animal models, particularly mice, hamsters, and non-human primates, were used to study the pathogenesis of COVID-19 [78]. By infecting animals with the virus, researchers have gained insights into how the virus spreads, replicates, and causes disease within the body. This knowledge has been critical for developing effective treatment strategies and understanding the virus' impact on different organs and tissues.

Yet, the morality of animal experimentation has long been contested. The case has been made that animals deserve ethical consideration and should not be subjected to unnecessary harm or suffering; conducting experiments on animals—as in the development of COVID-19 vaccines and treatments—has often involved procedures that may cause pain, distress, or discomfort [79].

The issue of whether animals are truly capable of suffering has long been debated in philosophy. One line of argumentation holds that since animals cannot communicate their experiences in human language, we cannot definitively know if they experience suffering in the same way humans do. The foundation for this argument is Descartes' view of animals as mechanistic beings devoid of consciousness or inner experiences [80, 81].

However, as Bentham famously countered, ""the question is not, can they reason? nor, can they talk? but, can they suffer" [18]? The burden of proof should be on those who deny animals' capacity to suffer, given the overwhelming evidence from neuroscience, ethology, and observational studies that suggest animals do experience pain, distress, and suffering in ways analogous to humans" [82–84].

What is truly at stake in this debate is not whether animals can suffer—the overwhelming majority of ethicists and scientists would agree that they do—, but rather, how shall we weigh human and non-human lives? What is our position as a species in the moral landscape vis-à-vis other species? Are human lives so valuable as to undermine the lives of non-human animals?

Consider this scenario: a trolley is bound to run over five gorillas who are tied to the tracks; the trolley can be diverted towards some tracks where one human is tied. Should the trolley be turned?

Interestingly, even some of the staunchest upholders of animal rights would seem to agree that, in this situation, it is better to save one human over five gorillas. For example, Tom Regan presents this famous thought experiment: "Imagine five survivors are on a lifeboat. Because of limits of size, the boat can only support four. All weigh approximately the same and would take up approximately the same amount of space. Four of the five are normal adult human beings. The fifth is a dog. One must be thrown overboard or else all will perish. Whom should it be" [85]? Regan argues the dog should be cast overboard, because "no reasonable person would suppose that the dog has a 'right to life' that is equal to the humans" [85]. But even if the dilemma came down to a large number of non-human animals, the decision ought to be the same: "a million dogs ought to be cast overboard if that is necessary to save the four normal humans" [85]. As Regan explains, the "harm that death is in the case of that animal is not as great a harm as the harm that death would be in the case of any of these humans" [85].

Now, why would the dog not have a right to life that is equal to the humans? It appears that Regan prefers average measures over total measures. As per his reasoning, to the extent that the human has more to gain in surviving than the dog, the human should be favored in the dilemma. Admittedly, on the average, a human has more fulfillment and joy than a dog. But the aggregate effect of the happiness of one million dogs would surely surpass the aggregate effect of the happiness of four humans. In the previous section I have already established that, despite the initial repugnance, in accounting for happiness total measures do seem more acceptable than average measures.

Therefore, some other principle must be sought in order to justify the preference to save one human over a greater number of non-human animals. Staunch defenders of animal rights insist that valuing human lives above non-human lives is a form of "speciesism." Peter Singer defines speciecists as those who "allow the interests of their own species to override the greater interests of members of other species" [86]. The premise of Singer is the principle of impartial beneficence, which I alluded to earlier in this chapter. As per this principle, it is inevitable to admit that Regan's decision is speciecist, as clearly, in his decision humans count for more and the interests of the human species override the greater interests of other species.

However, is it truly unethical to hold speciesist beliefs? Surely animals suffer. Yet, one could argue for justifiable speciesism not due to animals' lack of suffering but because of the unique obligations we hold towards our own species.

The concept of impartial beneficence appears logical within a theoretical realm and holds a commendable egalitarian dimension. If every individual is valued equally, it implies a certain degree of fairness for both the privileged and the underprivileged. Additionally, such impartial generosity serves as a foundation for combating favoritism and promoting a deeper sense of fairness.

Nevertheless, there are special obligations we owe to others, and there are situations where impartiality becomes impractical. Even staunch proponents of utilitarianism acknowledge this fact. Derek Parfit, for instance, illustrated this scenario: "Clare could either give her child some benefit, or give much greater benefits to some unfortunate stranger. Because she loves her child, she benefits him rather than the stranger" [51]. Parfit believed that, at worst, Clare engaged in some form of "blameless wrongdoing."

The general consensus tends to support the idea that parents have the right to prioritize their own children to some extent. Even William Godwin, a utilitarian philosopher from the 19th century who initially suggested he would prioritize saving an unrelated archbishop over his wife in a fire, eventually acknowledged the existence of special duties towards spouses and children [87]. If we acknowledge these exceptions within the family unit, could we not extend similar preferences to the broader human species?

If we acknowledge a mother's natural inclination to prioritize saving her own child over unrelated children, can't we similarly prioritize the welfare of our fellow human beings over non-human animals? Wouldn't this alignment be a true reflection of the essence of "humanism"? Just as a mother exhibits a bias, or "familyism," towards her own offspring, why shouldn't we display a similar bias, or "speciesism," towards our fellow human beings?

While some philosophers may recognize the strength of this argument, they may still express concerns regarding moral inconsistencies. Peter Singer, for instance, contends that speciesists are comparable to racists, who "violate the principle of equality by giving greater weight to the interests of members of their own race when there is a clash between their interests and the interests of those of another race... The pattern is identical in each case" [86].

However, it is debatable whether racism and speciesism can be equated in this manner. Unlike race, which is largely a social construct, the concept of family or species is not constructed in the same way. Throughout human history, societies have universally recognized families as fundamental units of social organization, and the distinction between humans and other species has been consistently acknowledged. In contrast, the notion of race is a relatively recent development, largely stemming from the historical context of the slave trade [88]. Therefore, concepts like family and species are more enduring and substantial, thereby providing firmer foundations for the notion of special obligations.

Some prominent animal advocates even recognize this. Consider Mary Midgley's words: "an emotional, rather than rational, preference for our own species is ... a necessary part of our social nature, in the same way that a preference for our own children is, and needs no more justification" [89]. Midgley argues for a type of speciesism based on preference, highlighting that it stems from our innate inclination towards favoring our own kind rather than any inherent inferiority of animals. This preference mirrors a mother's natural bond with her own offspring and is woven into our being, differing from prejudiced views based on race. Midgley explains: "the natural preference for one's own species does exist. It is not, like race-prejudice, a product of culture. It is found in all human cultures, and in cases of real competition it tends to operate very strongly" [89].

This form of speciesism would allow us to justify allocating healthcare resources to save human lives over non-human lives, even in hugely disproportionate numbers. After all, medicine is a humanistic practice, and that inevitably implies alleviating the suffering of our own species as a priority; concerns with other species are secondary.

But perhaps we have been considering the wrong trolley dilemma as an analogy. In using animals as subjects of experiments for our gain, we are not simply choosing whom to save from an already existing threat. Actually, we are using animals as means to our own ends, and to the extent that we subject them to the unpleasantness of experimentation, we are the very origin of the harm that falls upon them. In this regard, the relevant trolley scenario is akin to that of the fat man in the footbridge: a trolley is heading to run over five human beings, and a chimpanzee can be thrown from a footbridge so that its weight will stop the trolley and the lives of the humans will be saved; should the chimpanzee be thrown?

Now, it is interesting to note that research in moral psychology indicates that most people prefer saving humans over a larger number of non-human animals, if it comes down to simply diverting the trolley [90]. If it comes down to throwing the chimpanzee from the bridge, most people also agree that it is morally acceptable to do so. Interestingly, the dilemma has not been presented as throwing a non-human animal to save five humans, but rather, throwing a chimpanzee to save five chimpanzees; even in that case, most people approve of throwing the chimpanzee. If the intuition of most people is correct, then animals can indeed be used as means to an end, and animal experimentation may be justified.

Marc Hauser—the psychologist who has studied the dilemma of throwing one chimpanzee to save five chimpanzees—shares the same intuition, although he admits not fully understanding why it is acceptable to throw the chimpanzee from the bridge, but not to do the same with the fat man. His provisional answer is as follows: "Perhaps the difference stems instead from our emotional attachment, built over millions of years, designed to guarantee the welfare of humans but not other species. When faced with the trolley case, our emotional attachment to humans is greater than our attachment to animals, and thus our judgments shift" [91].

As in many other ethical dilemmas, some balancing act may be necessary. It is very hard to argue against the fact that animals have the capacity to suffer, and that implies that they have some rights. Yet, we have special obligations towards our own kind, and our greater attachment to humans is at least understandable. Nevertheless, our moral circle has been expanding over the centuries, and whereas gratuitous violence towards animals in the past was deemed acceptable, our current moral sensibilities preclude that.

We can certainly do more to alleviate human suffering, and that may even imply giving up eating meat altogether, as this would be a feasible project. Yet, at least for the time being, some experimentation with animals is still necessary to safeguard our safety as a species, and that was certainly the case during the management of the COVID-19 pandemic. As more pandemics are unfortunately bound to happen again, we will probably need to rely on animal experimentation again, and for that, we need to be prepared to challenge our conventional moral assumptions and reflect on our place in the moral landscape vis-à-vis non-human animals. While the necessity of moral experimentation will continue—and there will be probably moral justification to pursue it—, it is nevertheless true that some higher ethical standard must be placed, in order to make sure that experiments are done only when real scientific advantages are at stake, and proper steps are taken to maintain animal suffering at its possible minimum.

# References

1. Leavitt JW. Typhoid Mary: captive to the public's health. Beacon Press; 1997.
2. Wald P. Cultures and carriers: "Typhoid Mary" and the science of social control. Social Text. 1997;181–214.
3. Othman A, Darrow WW. The wall, the ban, and the objectification of women: Has "Uncle Sam" learned any lessons from "Typhoid Mary?" Int J Soc Qual. 2019;9:1–18.
4. Steere-Williams J. A "Menace" or a Martyr to the Public's health? Isis. 2020;111:818–21.
5. Ng BH, Nik Abeed NN, Abdul Hamid MF, Soo CI, Low HJ, Ban YA. What happens when we treat the "Typhoid Mary" of COVID-19. Respirology Case Rep. 2020;8: e00604.
6. Koh D. COVID-19 lockdowns throughout the world. Occup Med. 2020;70:322–322.
7. North Korea executes coronavirus patient for ditching quarantine. The Business Standard [Internet]. 2020 Feb 28 [cited 2024 Apr 22]; Available from: https://www.tbsnews.net/intern ational/coronavirus-chronicle/north-korea-executes-coronavirus-patient-ditching-quarantine.
8. Machiavelli N. Discourses on livy. University of Chicago Press; 2009.
9. Walzer M. Political action: the problem of dirty hands. Philos Public Aff. 1973;160–80.
10. Coady C. Dirty hands. In: Reading political philosophy: Machiavelli to Mill; 1993. p. 59–67.
11. Reverby SM. Tuskegee's truths: rethinking the Tuskegee syphilis study. UNC Press Books; 2012.

12. Brandt AM. Racism and research: the case of the Tuskegee Syphilis study. Hastings Center Rep. 1978;21–9.
13. Anscombe GE. Modern moral philosophy. In: The definition of morality. Routledge; 2020. p. 211–34.
14. Sprigge TL. A utilitarian reply to Dr. McCloskey. 1965.
15. Smart J. The methods of ethics and the methods of science. J Philos. 1965;62:344–9.
16. Laventhal N, Basak R, Dell ML, Diekema D, Elster N, Geis G, et al. The ethics of creating a resource allocation strategy during the COVID-19 pandemic. Pediatrics. 2020;146.
17. Taurek JM. Should the numbers count? Philos Public Aff. 1977;293–316.
18. Bentham J, Burns JH, Rosen F, Schofield P. The collected works of Jeremy Bentham. 1968;
19. Parfit D. Innumerate ethics. Philos Public Aff. 1978;285–301.
20. Norcross A. The scalar approach to utilitarianism. In: The Blackwell guide to Mill's utilitarianism; 2006. p. 217–32.
21. Sobel D. The impotence of the demandingness objection. Philos Imprint. 2007;7.
22. Nickel CH, Ruegg M, Pargger H, Bingisser R. Age, comorbidity, frailty status: effects on disposition and resource allocation during the COVID-19 pandemic. Swiss Med Wkly. 2020;150:w20269–w20269.
23. Montero-Odasso M, Hogan DB, Lam R, Madden K, MacKnight C, Molnar F, et al. Age alone is not adequate to determine health-care resource allocation during the COVID-19 pandemic. Can Geriatr J. 2020;23:152.
24. Neumann-Podczaska A, Al-Saad SR, Karbowski LM, Chojnicki M, Tobis S, Wieczorowska-Tobis K. COVID 19-clinical picture in the elderly population: a qualitative systematic review. Aging Dis. 2020;11:988.
25. Dai S-P, Zhao X, Wu J. Effects of comorbidities on the elderly patients with COVID-19: clinical characteristics of elderly patients infected with COVID-19 from sichuan, China. J Nutr Health Aging. 2021;25:18–24.
26. Bradley B. How bad is death? Can J Philos. 2007;37:111–27.
27. Glossary [Internet]. National Institute for Health and Care Excellence. [cited 2023 Jan 29]. Available from: https://www.nice.org.uk/glossary?letter=q#:~:text=One%20quality%2Dadjusted%20life%20year,a%200%20to%201%20scale.
28. Williams A. The value of QALYs. Health Soc Serv J. 1985;18.
29. Freath LL, Curry AS, Cork DM, Audhya IF, Gooch KL. QALYs and ambulatory status: societal preferences for healthcare decision making. J Med Econ. 2022;25:888–93.
30. Waring DR. Levels of benefit, utility scores and the QALY debate. In: Medical benefit and the human lottery: an egalitarian approach to patient selection; 2004. p. 99–114.
31. Rebeira M. QALYs and value assessment. Can Health Policy. 2022;2022:1–8.
32. Harris J. QALYfying the value of life. J Med Ethics. 1987;13:117–23.
33. Zwolinski M. The separateness of persons and liberal theory. J Value Inquiry. 2008;42:147.
34. Voorhoeve A, Fleurbaey M. Egalitarianism and the separateness of persons. Utilitas. 2012;24:381–98.
35. Brink D. The separateness of persons, distributive norms, and moral theory. Value, Welfare, Morality. 1993;252–89.
36. Rawls J. A theory of justice. Cambridge, MA, US: Harvard University Press; 1971.
37. Yudkowsky E. Torture versus Dust Specks [Internet]. Less Wrong. 2007 [cited 2024 Apr 30]. Available from: https://www.lesswrong.com/posts/3wYTFWY3LKQCnAptN/torture-vs-dust-specks.
38. Scanlon TM. What we owe to each other. Harvard University Press; 2000.
39. Caselli F, Grigoli F, Lian W, Sandri D. The great lockdown: dissecting the economic effects. World Econ Outlook. 2020;65:84.
40. Onyeaka H, Anumudu CK, Al-Sharify ZT, Egele-Godswill E, Mbaegbu P. COVID-19 pandemic: a review of the global lockdown and its far-reaching effects. Sci Prog. 2021;104:00368504211019854.
41. Melnick ER, Ioannidis JP. Should governments continue lockdown to slow the spread of covid-19? BMJ. 2020;369.

42. Kamm F. Moral Reasoning in a Pandemic. Boston Review [Internet]. 2020 Jul 6 [cited 2024 Apr 30]; Available from: https://www.bostonreview.net/articles/f-m-kamm-tk/.

43. Norcross A. Contractualism and aggregation. Soc Theory Pract. 2002;28:303–14.

44. Shafi S, Gentilello L. A nationwide speed limit ≤65 miles per hour will save thousands of lives. Am J Surg. 2007;193:719–22.

45. Vadeby A. How many lives could be saved if everyone complied with the speed limit?–a case study from Sweden. Transp Res Procedia. 2023;72:3024–30.

46. Norcross A. Great harms from small benefits grow: how death can be outweighed by headaches. Analysis. 1998;58:152–8.

47. Boltuc P. Moral neighborhoods. Dialogue Universalism. 2001;11.

48. Cottingham J. Caring at a distance:(Im) partiality, moral motivation and the ethics of representation-partiality, distance and moral obligation. Ethics, Place Environ. 2000;3:309–13.

49. Ashford E. Utilitarianism, integrity, and partiality. J Philos. 2000;97:421–39.

50. Singer P. Famine, affluence, and morality. In: Applied ethics. Routledge; 2017. p. 132–42.

51. Parfit D. Reasons and persons. OUP Oxford; 1984.

52. Johnson BL, Lichtveld MY. Environmental policy and public health. CRC Press; 2017.

53. Roberts MA. The existence puzzles: an introduction to population ethics. Oxford University Press; 2024.

54. Narveson J. Moral problems of population. Monist. 1973;62–86.

55. Arrhenius G. The impossibility of a satisfactory population ethics. In: Descriptive and normative approaches to human behavior. World Scientific; 2012. p. 1–26.

56. Caviola L, Althaus D, Mogensen AL, Goodwin GP. Population ethical intuitions. Cognition. 2022;218: 104941.

57. Broome J. Should we value population?*. 2005;

58. Benatar D. Better never to have been: the harm of coming into existence. OUP Oxford; 2006.

59. Schell J. The fate of the Earth and the abolition: and, the abolition. Stanford University Press; 2000.

60. Finneron-Burns E. What's wrong with human extinction? Can J Philos. 2017;47:327–43.

61. MacAskill W. Longtermism [Internet]. [cited 2024 May 1]. Available from: https://www.wil liammacaskill.com/longtermism#:~:text=Longtermism%20is%20based%20on%20the,or% 20poorly%20their%20lives%20go.

62. Bostrom N. Existential risks: analyzing human extinction scenarios and related hazards. J Evol Technol. 2002;9.

63. Balfour D. Pascal's mugger strikes again. Utilitas. 2021;33:118–24.

64. Bostrom N. Pascal's mugging. Analysis. 2009;69:443–5.

65. Malthus TR. An essay on the principle of population: or, a view of its past and present effects on human happiness, with an inquiry into our prospects respecting the future removal or mitigation of the evils which it occasions. London: Reeves and Turner; 1878.

66. Price D. Of population and false hopes: Malthus and his legacy. Popul Environ. 1998;19:205–19.

67. Stokstad E. Will Malthus continue to be wrong? Science. 2005;309:102–102.

68. Smith P. Malthus is still wrong: we can feed a world of 9–10 billion, but only by reducing food demand. Proc Nutr Soc. 2015;74:187–90.

69. Pressman M. A defence of average utilitarianism. Utilitas. 2015;27:389–424.

70. Qizilbash M. The mere addition paradox, parity and vagueness. Philos Phenomenol Res. 2007;75:129–51.

71. Temkin LS. Intransitivity and the mere addition paradox. Philos Public Aff. 1987;138–87.

72. Temkin LS. Lessons to be learned from the Mere addition paradox. In: The Oxford Handbook of Population Ethics; 2022. p. 161.

73. Fan C, Wu Y, Rui X, Yang Y, Ling C, Liu S, et al. Animal models for COVID-19: advances, gaps and perspectives. Signal Transduct Target Ther. 2022;7:220.

74. Muñoz-Fontela C, Dowling WE, Funnell SG, Gsell P-S, Riveros-Balta AX, Albrecht RA, et al. Animal models for COVID-19. Nature. 2020;586:509–15.

75. Caldera-Crespo LA, Paidas MJ, Roy S, Schulman CI, Kenyon NS, Daunert S, et al. Experimental models of COVID-19. Front Cell Infect Microbiol. 2022;11: 792584.
76. Vanderslott S, Palmer A, Thomas T, Greenhough B, Stuart A, Henry JA, et al. Co-producing human and animal experimental subjects: exploring the views of UK COVID-19 vaccine trial participants on animal testing. Sci Technol Human Values. 2023;48:909–37.
77. Moothedath M, Muhamood M, Bhosale YS, Bhatia A, Gupta P, Reddy MRH, et al. COVID and animal trials: a systematic review. J Pharm Bioallied Sci. 2021;13:S31–5.
78. Hansur L, Louisa M, Wuyung PE. Approach for the study of COVID-19 infection and vaccine development using mice model: a narrative review. AIP Publishing; 2022.
79. Francione GL, Garner R. The animal rights debate: abolition or regulation? Columbia University Press; 2010.
80. Cottingham J. A Brute to the Brutes?': descartes. Treat Animals Philos. 1978;53:551–9.
81. Rollin BE. Animal pain: what it is and why it matters. J Ethics. 2011;15:425–37.
82. Simpson J. Non-human animals feel pain in a morally relevant sense. Philosophia. 2023;51:329–36.
83. Dawkins MS. The science of animal suffering. Ethology. 2008;114:937–45.
84. Singer P. All animals are equal. Appl Ethics: Crit Concepts Philos. 1989;4:51–79.
85. Regan T. The case for animal rights. Los Angeles: University of California Press; 2004.
86. Singer P. Animal liberation. New York: Open Road; 2015.
87. Godwin W. An enquiry concerning political justice. OUP Oxford; 2013.
88. Davis DB. Constructing race: a reflection. William Mary Q. 1997;54:7–18.
89. Midgley M. Animals and why they matter. University of Georgia Press; 1984.
90. Petrinovich L, O'Neill P, Jorgensen M. An empirical study of moral intuitions: toward an evolutionary ethics. J Pers Soc Psychol. 1993;64:467.
91. Hauser M. Moral minds: how nature designed our universal sense of right and wrong. Ecco/HarperCollins Publishers; 2006.

# Conclusion

**Abstract** This section presents three main conclusions. Firstly, voluntary active euthanasia may be considered compassionate despite distinctions between causing and allowing harm. Secondly, abortion may be morally permissible, especially in the first trimester when a fetus is not considered a person. Lastly, in public health decisions, numerical considerations are important, and total utilitarianism may be more appropriate than average utilitarianism. While trolley scenarios aid in refining moral intuitions in medical ethics, they have limitations in capturing the complexities of real-life moral decision-making.

After this extensive consideration of trolley dilemmas, I can now reach three tentative sets of conclusions. First, there may be relevant moral distinctions between doing and allowing harm, but that does not imply that voluntary active euthanasia is always immoral; in fact, sometimes it would be the compassionate procedure to follow.

Second, a fetus in the first trimester is not a person, and therefore, in those cases there should be no moral opposition to abortion. Potentiality does not grant an entity personhood, although I acknowledge that in the grand scheme of things, the interest of future people does count. Abortion may also be morally acceptable on the grounds of self-defense and intrinsic women's rights, although late-term abortions for trivial reasons do at least seem unvirtuous, albeit not necessarily morally prohibited.

Third, in making decisions in the realm of public health, numbers do matter, although it is not clear what the best counting criterion is. In this context, as stated above, future generations count, and that may entail bringing about a much larger population size than most people are prepared to accept. Likewise, it is sensible to accept that animals suffer pain, but it also seems reasonable to posit that we have special obligations towards the wellbeing of our own human species, and if that entails using animals in very narrow lines of biomedical research, we must be prepared to bite that bullet.

In coming to these conclusions, I have used trolley scenarios and other thought experiments. The purpose of this has been to test our moral intuitions as to what moral principles are the most adequate. But can we really be sure that testing moral intuitions tells us something relevant about the ethical adequacy of particular actions?

© The Author(s) 2024

G. Andrade, *Trolleyology in Medicine*, SpringerBriefs in Ethics, https://doi.org/10.1007/978-3-031-72806-8

Trolley dilemmas are central to moral psychology, but can we make the leap towards normative theory?

Many philosophers have struggled with this question. In the 18th Century, David Hume famously framed the problem as follows: "the distinction of vice and virtue is not founded merely on the relations of objects, nor is perceived by reason" [1]. In Hume's reasoning, it is not possible to derive a normative statement from a descriptive statement. It is one thing to say how the world is, and quite another to say how it ought to be.

Trolley dilemmas tell us what most people think about morality, but does it tell us whether those ideas reflect the real distinction between right and wrong? Ultimately, no. Nevertheless, trolley dilemmas do serve a moral goal. As with any other thought scenario (or "intuition pump", as some philosophers call them), trolley dilemmas serve a clarifying purpose, but they can never be the sole (or even ultimate) guide to morality.

In the context of medical ethics, we can think of trolley dilemmas as tools to refine our thinking. In this endeavor, we can follow Daniel Dennet's enlightening metaphor: "A tool wielded well becomes almost as much a part of you as your hands and feet, and this is especially true of tools for thinking. Equipped with these simple all-purpose thinking tools, you can approach the difficult explorations ahead with sharper senses: you can see an opening, hear a warning bell, smell a rat, or feel a misstep that you might well miss without their help" [2]. But Dennett is also quick to mention that "thinking tools are also weapons, and the imagery of combat is appropriate", [2] to the extent that they may be irresponsibly used by combatants who want to merely score points with little regard to intellectual honesty. As Dennet explains, "in the heat of battle even great thinkers can resort to dirty tricks in their eagerness to get you to see things their way, and constructive criticism can quickly shade into ridicule when an opportunity to launch a zinger arises" [2].

Trolley scenarios may serve to clarify our moral intuitions, but they can be quite unrealistic. They can be criticized for presenting overly simplified scenarios that do not accurately reflect the complexity of real-life moral decisions. In real-world situations, there are usually more factors to consider than just pulling a lever to divert a trolley. These dilemmas often evoke emotional responses from us, but these responses may not accurately reflect how we would behave in similar real-world situations. The hypothetical nature of the dilemmas can lead to a sense of emotional detachment that does not capture the complexity of moral decision-making in practice.

Furthermore, as we have seen, these dilemmas offer only two options, forcing us to choose between sacrificing one life to save many or doing nothing and allowing many to die. However, real-life moral decisions often involve a wider range of possible actions and consequences. A related problem is that in trolley dilemmas we do not face any real consequences for our decisions, which can make it easier to make a choice without fully considering the moral implications.

We can still acknowledge these limitations without needing to throw the baby out with the bathwater, especially in the context of medical ethics. Thinking about euthanasia, abortion or the intricacies of decisions in public health is a difficult task, and by no means our moral decision-making in this realm should be left off entirely to the dictum of intuitions in highly artificial scenarios about trolleys running over people. But certainly, such scenarios help medical practitioners to be better prepared when facing tough moral decisions.

In a way, trolley dilemmas work as dummies in clinical training. Practicing with a rubber simulated patient will never teach medical students the entirety of what needs to be known in order to become a successful clinician. But such resources are still of great importance in medical education.

Medical ethics is a messy business with many confounding factors. Consequently, although it is likely true that one cannot derive an "ought" from an "is", we still need some scientific approach in order to arrive at sound moral decision-making in medicine. Very much as scientists work in experiments in order to isolate confounding factors, those engaged in medical ethics must find some way of assessing the core elements of particular ethical situations. In this regard, trolley scenarios provide a good service. Frances Kamm explains it as follows: "real-life cases have a lot of factors going on, and it's hard to test whether it's this factor that's crucial or that factor. You have to artificially construct cases to focus on the factors that are important. It's like the scientist in the lab who has to figure out whether, say, the dust particle makes a difference to friction, and tries to hold everything else constant" [3].

Ultimately, while trolley dilemmas offer valuable insights into moral intuitions and serve as tools for refining ethical thinking in medicine, they are but one aspect of a complex landscape. Recognizing their limitations, we must approach medical ethics with a nuanced understanding that extends beyond hypothetical scenarios. Trolley scenarios are scientifically inspired to the extent that they aid in isolating crucial factors for moral analysis. Yet, in navigating the intricate terrain of medical ethics, a comprehensive approach blending scientific inquiry with ethical reflection—especially on a case-by-case basis—remains indispensable for sound moral decision-making.

# References

1. Hume D. A treatise of human nature. Oxford University Press; 2000.
2. Dennett DC. Intuition pumps and other tools for thinking. WW Norton & Company; 2013.
3. Edmonds D. Matters of life and death [Internet]. Prospect. 2010 [cited 2024 May 3]. Available from: https://www.prospectmagazine.co.uk/essays/54491/matters-of-life-and-death

© The Author(s) 2024
G. Andrade, *Trolleyology in Medicine*, SpringerBriefs in Ethics,
https://doi.org/10.1007/978-3-031-72806-8